FRONTIERS IN PAIN RESEARCH

Frontiers in Pain Research

Alexandre Lucas
Editor

Nova Science Publishers, Inc.
New York

For permission to use material from this book please contact us:
Telephone 631-231-7269; Fax 631-231-8175
Web Site: http://www.novapublishers.com

LIBRARY OF CONGRESS CATALOGING-IN-PUBLICATION DATA
Frontiers in pain research / Alexandre Lucas, editor.
p. ; cm.
Includes bibliographical references and index.
ISBN 1-59454-828-5
1. Pain. 2. Pain--Treatment. I. Lucas, Alexandre.
[DNLM: 1. Pain--etiology. 2. Pain--therapy. WL 704 F935 2005]
RB127.F79 2005
616'.0472--dc22 2005034375

Published by Nova Science Publishers, Inc. ✦ New York

CONTENTS

PREFACE

Extant research suggests that pain, especially chronic pain (i.e., lasting 3 months or more) may be an important factor in seeking medical care. Pain symptoms are commonly experienced in the general population of adults and children, as well as chronically-ill populations including persons living with human immunodeficiency virus (HIV). Moreover, there is considerable evidence that pain has an adverse impact on health-related quality of life (HRQOL) in these populations. Nevertheless, the relationship between pain and utilization of health services is not well-understood. Chapter one draws together evidence from diverse populations to highlight those factors that have been shown to modulate the association between pain and health care use, including complementary and alternative medicine (CAM) approaches, as well as conventional medical care. These factors are discussed within the conceptual framework of Andersen's Behavioral Model of Health Services Use, which holds that contextual (i.e., community and environmental factors) and individual predisposing, enabling, and need characteristics influence use of health services. Predisposing characteristics are based on the proposition that factors such as age, sex, and race/ethnicity affect an individual's propensity to use different types of health services although these conditions are not directly responsible for use. Enabling characteristics include the economic and social resources that facilitate or impede care. Need-related characteristics refer to the presence or severity of illness. Pain is thus properly viewed as a perceived need characteristic within this framework as it is assessed by the individual experiencing the pain. Special attention in this chapter is paid to specific need factors such as psychological distress as well as drug and/or alcohol abuse that, in conjunction with pain, may impact use of medical care. The chapter also details future research directions. Current conceptualizations view pain as a multidimensional construct incorporating social, psychological/behavioral, and physiological aspects, and thus further study is needed to better understand how these individual, yet related aspects of pain might interact with other characteristics within the Andersen Model in determining health services use. In addition, future investigations should examine whether alleviating pain symptoms leads to decreased use of health services. Through improved management of pain, it may be possible to reduce health services utilization among persons experiencing pain and thus decrease health expenditures while also improving their HRQOL.

The pain experience includes a sensory-discriminative and an emotional-affective component. The sensory dimension describes the quality, intensity, and spatio-temporal characteristics of the sensation. The affective dimension refers to the unpleasantness or aversion of sensation. The great progress at the genetic, molecular, cellular, and systemic level on the study of the sensory dimension of pain has been made over the past four decades. However, "*to consider only the sensory features of pain, and ignore its motivational and affective properties, is to look at only part of the problem and not even the must important part of that"* [107]. A line of clinic observations indicate that the patients with chronic pain suffer from much more affective disturbance than pain itself. Obviously, physiological arousal and hypervigilance to pain cause negative affect, such as anxiety, anger, worry, aversion, even tendency of suicide, these negative affective states in turn enhance pain sensation. Today, more and more attention has been paid to the study on mechanisms underlying affective dimension of pain. In order to deepen and expand our understanding of the nature of pain, chapter two summarizes the main progress and recent findings from our laboratory regarding the affective component of pain in neuroanatomy, neurophysiology, and cell biochemistry.

Clinical observations have shown that wide variations in response to analgesics exist. Some individuals exhibit unrelieved pain despite high doses and others exhibit side effects even with low doses. The effectiveness and side effects of analgesics may be related to the dose, route, and time of administration, as well as genetic factors that may predispose individual variations in response to pain and analgesics. Several studies have examined the rhythms of various types of pain and neuropeptides associated with pain. Chapter three will review evidence from the literature, including human and animal studies, that suggests that variations in response to pain and analgesics may be explained by rhythmic, pharmacokinetic, and genetic factors that affect the metabolism of and response to analgesics. There will be two major sections to the chapter: 1) Rhythmic variations in mechanisms involved in pain and analgesia and 2) Pharmacokinetic variations in metabolism and disposition of analgesics. Both of these sections will discuss genetic factors that may influence individual responses to pain and analgesics. The roles of these variations need to be thoroughly investigated. Theoretically, potential development of analgesics and individualized dosage regimens for patients with pain may be based on these variations.

Despite years of research and available medications, pain remains one of the most under-treated medical conditions. This is due, in part, to the complexity and heterogeneity of the condition itself. Both clinical and preclinical studies indicate that pain resulting from different etiologies develops and is maintained via differing biological processes. Pragmatically, this has culminated in the use of targeted analgesics, i.e. medications efficacious in and individually approved for only certain subtypes of pain. However, the desire to create non-opioid broad-spectrum analgesics remains as the treatment of pain would be greatly simplified if physicians did not have to tailor medication to each individual patient. Additionally, developing a broad-spectrum analgesic with an improved safety profile is paramount so that physicians and patients would not have to try to find the often inadequate but acceptable balance between moderate efficacy and tolerable side effects. Nicotinic acetylcholine receptor (nAChR) agonists have the potential to be broad-spectrum analgesics based on preclinical studies demonstrating efficacy in numerous pain states including multiple forms of acute, chronic, inflammatory and neuropathic pain. Intriguingly, research indicates that the exact mechanism(s) through which nAChR agonists induce analgesia may differ depending upon the type of pain, thus further supporting the contention that these compounds may have the appropriate biological properties to relieve a wide range of clinical pain states. However, given the ubiquitous distribution of nAChRs and the number of biological functions modulated by the nAChR system, achieving adequate pain relief without adverse side effects remains the greatest challenge. Chapter four will review the current understanding of pain states with regard to the development of broad-spectrum analgesics, using nAChR agonists as an example of the promise and challenges inherent in this approach.

In 1965 Melzak and Wall gate control theory proposed that stimulation of A-beta fibers modulates the dorsal horn "gate" and therefore reduces the nociceptive input from periphery. The gate control theory sparked clinician's interest, and already, by 1967, Shealy and colleagues published the first report on spinal cord stimulation (SCS) in humans. The first SCS was placed intrathecaly via open laminotomy. Although effective in many patients, the underdeveloped hardware significantly slowed down the progress of SCS in the 1970's. With significant improvement in hardware design and simplifaction of trial techniques with introducing epidural approach in 1980's, the SCS gained in popularity and now is routinely used in clinical practice to treat many chronic pain conditions.

Over the last two decades, many clinical outcome studies have supported the use of SCS for chronic pain. The SCS is particularly beneficial in reducing pain in patients with lumbar and cervical radiculopathy and complex regional pain syndrome (CRPS). Several randomized studies have shown the clear advantages of SCS over re-operation in patients who failed back surgery. Recently, there is good evidence that SCS may be very beneficial for treatment of chest pain due to coronary artery disease in patients who fail conservative treatment options.

Over the last two decades, the understanding of SCS mechanisms of action evolved significantly, which is discussed in chapter five. Rather than explained by gate control theory, it seems that mechanisms of SCS action are more complex. These mechanisms may involve increased dorsal horn inhibitory action of GABA, adenosine and the disinhibition of descending analgesia pathways originating in periaqueductal gray (PAG). Due to these modulatory actions in the CNS, the SCS is often named "Neuromodulation." The history of SCS development is a perfect example of how new ideas can spark expansion of useful clinical application.

Studies in animals have shown that cortical representations of sensory surfaces reorganize after peripheral deafferentation so that some of the deprived cortex comes to be activated by inputs from skin regions near the deafferented zone. These changes may occur rapidly (short-term changes) or they may become progressively more pronounced over time (long-term changes). These changes of receptive fields are not confined to the cortex but also occur in the spinal dorsal horn and brainstem structures of the somatosensory system (for example in the cuneatus nucleus). Changes in subcortical structures could be one of the mechanisms subserving large scale reorganization in primary somatosensory cortex (S1). In humans, neurophysiologic techniques including magnetoencefalography (MEG), somatosensory evoked potentials (SEPs) and laser evoked potentials (LEPs) have been used to demonstrate aspects of short-tem and long-terms changes in the S1 and in subcortical structures in different conditions: i) in subjects after peripheral acute or chronic deafferentation; ii) in amputee patients with phantom limb pain and non-painful sensations; iii) in patients with chronic pain without massive large-fibres deafferentation; iiii) in normal subjects in whom pain was induced experimentally. All these studies examined in chapter six lead to the conclusion that pathological perturbations of somatic input may induce major neuroplastic changes at different levels of the Central Nervous System in humans and that pain is crucial in promoting reorganization in both somatosensory and nociceptive systems.

The relationship between the cingulum and the processing of emotions was first established by Papez in the 1930's. Since then, many studies have related the cingulum bundle to areas of the limbic system that constitute a circuit which includes the hippocampus, the mamillary bodies, the anterior thalamic nucleus and the cingulate cortex. Some studies have associated limbic structures with cognitive and affective pain processing. For more than four decades, the cingulotomy has been used in the treatment of patients with central or intractable pain or who exhibit refractority to pharmacological treatment to pain. Recent findings including those of functional image studies highlight the activation of limbic structures such as the thalamus, anterior cingulate cortex (ACC), insular cortex and mesolimbic dopaminergic nuclei in central pain processing. This evidence makes relevant the animal experimental study of loci, pathways, neurotransmitters and receptors regarding the relationship between the limbic system and chronic central neuropathic pain. The experiments were performed based on the somatic inflammatory process (hind paw carrageenan injection) and peripheral denervation (thermonociception prior to sciatic transection), both which trigger quantifiable chronic nociception that is expressed either as autotomy behaviour (AB) or self injury behaviour (SIB).

The results have shown that the electrical stimulation of the cingulum bundle simultaneously to an inflammatory painful process accelerates the onset and enhances the rate of autotomy induced by hind paw carrageenan injections. Moreover, an electrical stimulation of the anteriomedial and mediodorsal thalamic nuclei, which is the origin of the cingulum bundle and whose glutamatergic afferents have been widely described, also enhances incidence and shorten onset as well as increase intensity of AB. In chapter seven, the memory mechanisms associated with the ACC and related to their consolidation will also be reviewed. In this matter, AB is susceptible of being diminished by a muscarinic blockade of cholinergic transmission using scopolamine.

Childbirth provides the paradoxical circle of both pain and joy with physical, emotional, cognitive, and spiritual dimensions. Complex factors influence childbirth pain. Chapter eight reports on two decades of qualitative cross cultural studies of childbearing women and a review of the literature focusing on attitudes, perceptions, and meaning of the pain associated with giving birth, pain related behaviors, coping mechanisms for dealing with childbirth pain, and management of the pain of childbirth. Implications for clinical practice and future research are identified.

In Frontiers in Pain Research
Editor: Alexendre Lucas, pp.1-26

ISBN 1-59454-828-5

Chapter 1

PAIN AND UTILIZATION OF HEALTH SERVICES

Jennie C. I. Tsao

UCLA Pediatric Pain Program, Department of Pediatrics, David Geffen School of Medicine at UCLA

Aram Dobalian

VA Greater Los Angeles Center of Excellence for the Study of Healthcare Provider Behavior, Sepulveda Ambulatory Care Center and Nursing Home, and UCLA Department of Health Services, School of Public Health

Lonnie K. Zeltzer

UCLA Pediatric Pain Program, Departments of Pediatrics, Anesthesiology, Psychiatry and Biobehavioral Sciences, David Geffen School of Medicine at UCLA.

ABSTRACT

Extant research suggests that pain, especially chronic pain (i.e., lasting 3 months or more) may be an important factor in seeking medical care. Pain symptoms are commonly experienced in the general population of adults and children, as well as chronically-ill populations including persons living with human immunodeficiency virus (HIV). Moreover, there is considerable evidence that pain has an adverse impact on health-related quality of life (HRQOL) in these populations. Nevertheless, the relationship between pain and utilization of health services is not well-understood. This chapter draws together evidence from diverse populations to highlight those factors that have been shown to modulate the association between pain and health care use, including complementary and alternative medicine (CAM) approaches, as well as conventional medical care. These factors are discussed within the conceptual framework of Andersen's Behavioral Model of Health Services Use, which holds that contextual (i.e., community and environmental factors) and individual predisposing, enabling, and need characteristics influence use of health services. Predisposing characteristics are based on the proposition that factors such as age, sex, and race/ethnicity affect an individual's propensity to use different types of health services although these conditions are not directly responsible for use. Enabling characteristics include the economic and social resources that facilitate or impede care. Need-related characteristics refer to the presence or severity of illness. Pain is thus properly viewed as a perceived need characteristic within this framework as it is assessed by the individual experiencing the pain. Special attention in this chapter is paid to specific need factors such as psychological distress as well as drug and/or alcohol abuse that, in conjunction with pain, may impact use of medical care. The chapter also details future research directions. Current conceptualizations view pain as a multidimensional construct incorporating social, psychological/behavioral, and physiological aspects, and thus further study is needed to better understand how these individual, yet related aspects of pain might interact with other characteristics within the Andersen Model in determining health services use. In addition, future investigations should examine whether alleviating pain symptoms leads to decreased use of health services. Through improved management of pain, it may be possible to reduce health services utilization among persons experiencing pain and thus decrease health expenditures while also improving their HRQOL.

INTRODUCTION

The purpose of this chapter is to present trends and summarize research and policy issues related to the role of pain in the use of personal health services. Most of the research discussed in this chapter are concerned with the role of chronic pain (defined in various ways), rather than acute pain, in the use of health services. Chronic pain is defined by the International Association for the Study of Pain (IASP) as continuous or recurrent pain that persists for longer than the normal time of healing, generally about three months.[1] However, the required duration for pain to be considered chronic varies by health condition and can be as little as one month. Furthermore, some pain specialists continue to classify chronic pain under a prior definition which required pain to persist for longer than six months in order to be considered chronic. In contrast, acute pain is usually of brief duration and the intensity of that pain tends to decrease after healing begins. Acute pain may result from injury, surgery, illness, or other identifiable cause. The failure to properly treat acute pain can delay recovery and may lead to the development of chronic pain.

Few studies have specifically examined pain within the broader context of access to health services. Nevertheless, the importance of pain in care-seeking behavior has been recognized for some time. For example, Von Korff and colleagues (1991)[2] noted that chronic pain conditions are among the most common reasons for seeking health care, particularly ambulatory care.[3] However, as Von Korff et al. discussed, it does not necessarily follow that persons with chronic pain consume larger amounts of health care than those without chronic pain. Rather, the high frequency of health care visits for chronic pain may simply reflect a high prevalence of such pain conditions in the general population rather than above average rates of health care utilization by persons with chronic pain. To better understand the prevalence and importance of pain in access to health care, researchers have conducted large-scale epidemiologic studies of pain in the general population within a number of developed nations. The findings of these studies are discussed below.

In order to understand the role of pain in health services utilization, it is helpful to consider the myriad factors that may also influence whether an individual chooses to access health care. For purposes of this chapter, access to health services is defined as the factors that influence entry into the health care system or the use of health care. Researchers have proposed various models for understanding why a person uses health care, but most models of access to health care are based on either a psychological[4] or sociological framework. The Health Belief Model, a primarily psychologically-based model, posits that the use of health services is determined by an individual's beliefs about disease (i.e. the individual's susceptibility to the disease and its seriousness) and the effectiveness of the health care system to prevent or treat disease. Demographic variables such as the person's age and sex, psychological variables such as personality and peer group pressure, and structural variables such as knowledge of the disease and prior experience with it all are factors that modify the likelihood of seeking care. Cues to action such as mass media campaigns that are designed to heighten awareness of a particular disease or of risk factors associated with the disease also influence how an individual perceives the threat of a particular disease, and thus whether the person chooses to seek care. In this model, pain influences how serious a "disease" is perceived to be, although pain may also act as a barrier to action if, for example, the treatment is likely to be painful. The Health Beliefs Model is sometimes criticized for not adequately considering cultural factors and socioeconomic status.

Andersen's Behavioral Model of Health Services Use, one commonly used conceptual framework for understanding utilization of health services, is based on a systems perspective, and considers both contextual and individual characteristics as important factors that influence whether an individual accesses care.[5] Within this framework, contextual factors include aspects of the health care organizations, the health care providers, and the community. In contrast, individual characteristics are specific to a particular person, including, for example, the person's age and the type of health insurance plan in which the individual is enrolled.

According to the current Behavioral Model of Health Services Use, both contextual and individual characteristics are divided into three components: predisposing, enabling, and need characteristics.[6, 7] By contextual, the model refers to aggregate level community and environmental factors. Individual factors include characteristics that are specific to the person. Predisposing characteristics are based on the proposition that factors such as age, sex, and race/ethnicity influence an individual's propensity to use different types of health services although these conditions are not directly responsible for use. Contextual predisposing characteristics would include, for example, the age and sex makeup of a community since the availability of different types of health care organizations and health care providers is dependent on the demographic makeup of that community. Enabling characteristics include the economic and social resources at either the individual or contextual levels that facilitate or impede care, and include, for example, health insurance coverage and whether an individual has a usual source of health care. Need characteristics refer to the presence or severity of illness, as assessed by both laypersons (perceived need) and health care providers (evaluated need). Contextual need characteristics include, for example, health-related measures of the environment such as air quality. Within this conceptual framework, pain would be an individual perceived need characteristic, as pain is an aspect of how people view their health and functional status. Ultimately, it is the need characteristics that are recognized by the layperson as sufficient to require medical care.

This conceptual framework for understanding the myriad factors that impact the use of medical care provides the context within which research concerning the role of pain in the use of health services is discussed in this chapter. The chapter is subdivided by population type and begins with the largest body of work which is focused on the general population of adults, followed by sections devoted to children and special populations, including persons living with human immunodeficiency virus (HIV) and veterans. For each population, the section begins with a summary of the epidemiologic studies of the prevalence of pain symptoms with a focus on chronic pain and explores demographic factors related to increased likelihood of self-reported pain. This is followed by a discussion of the extant research on the role of pain in the use of various health services, including complementary and alternative medicine (CAM) approaches where such studies exist. In addition, the impact of comorbid psychological symptoms and pain on health services use is discussed. Important considerations specific to the study of pain and health services use in children and special populations are also highlighted within these sections. The chapter concludes with a discussion of future research directions that would lead to a greater understanding of the relationship between pain and health services utilization.

Chronic Pain in the General Population

Epidemologic Findings

Relatively few studies have examined the prevalence of pain complaints in the general adult population. In an early study, Frolund and Frolund (1986)[8] reported that pain was a major reason for medical consultation with 22% of all health care contacts due to pain. These authors also reported that the proportion of medical visits for acute and chronic pain was 61% and 39%, respectively. More recently, Verhaak and colleagues (1998)[9] reviewed 15 studies on the prevalence of benign chronic pain at the population or primary care level in respondents aged 18 to 75 years. As these authors pointed out, the term "benign" is rarely mentioned explicitly in such studies but was used to select epidemiological works that examined pain, as long as the study was not exclusively focused on acute pain or on pain as a consequence of a clearly defined disease such as cancer or rheumatoid arthritis. Notably, the studies reviewed spanned several countries: the United States (U.S.) (4 studies), the United Kingdom (U.K.) (3 studies), Denmark (2 studies), Sweden (2 studies), Canada, Finland, Germany, and New Zealand (1 study each). Verhaak et al. reported that estimates of the prevalence of chronic pain ranged between 2%[10] and 40%,[11] with the median being 15%.

Although the methods used to assess pain varied across studies and included telephone surveys, postal questionnaires, interviews and general practitioner assessments, Verhaak et al. (1998)[9] found that the differences in prevalence rates could not be explained by variations due to the methodology used. Similarly, despite differences in definitions of chronicity across studies (i.e., ranging from less than 1 month to greater than 6 months), prevalence estimates were not greatly impacted by variations in the time period used to define chronic pain. Some studies employed a graded approach to defining chronic pain (i.e., assessing dimensions such as severity and persistence) whereas others relied on a more simplified measure of chronic pain (e.g., pain present vs. absent). However, these approaches yielded similar results. The studies that used the more complex, graded definition of chronic pain evidenced a median prevalence rate of 13.5%, compared to those that employed a simpler definition which yielded a median prevalence rate of 16%. Based on these data, the authors concluded that a cautious estimate of a 10% prevalence rate for chronic pain in the general population was indicated.

Regarding patients' sociodemographic characteristics, there was more consensus across studies.[9] In seven of the 15 studies, chronic pain was more prevalent among women than men; in two studies prevalence rates were similar across sex. Prevalence was found to generally increase with age, and some studies reported peak prevalence between the ages of 45 and 65 years. Lower income groups had higher prevalence rates. The most common pain complaint was musculoskeletal pain (back pain, neck pain, shoulder pain), with headaches and abdominal pain also frequently mentioned.

Since the review by Verhaak et al. (1998)[9], at least three studies have been published examining the prevalence of chronic pain in the general population. Chrubasik and colleagues (1998)[12], using a postal survey, reported a 40% prevalence rate for prolonged pain in a German population sample. Their findings are consistent with at least two prior studies, both included in the Verhaak et al. review, one conducted in Sweden[11] and the other in the U.S.[13]. Supporting the findings of Verhaak and colleagues, Chrubasik et al. also found that older age and being female were associated with increased pain prevalence. A more recent study conducted by Blyth et al. (2001)[14] in Australia using a telephone survey, reported that the prevalence of chronic pain was 17.1% in men and 20.0% in women. The authors also found that older age, female sex, having lower levels of education and not having private health insurance were significantly associated with having chronic pain. In addition, having chronic pain was also strongly associated with receiving disability or unemployment benefits, being unemployed for health reasons, having poor self-rated health, and high levels of psychological distress. The authors concluded that chronic pain impacts a large proportion of the adult working age population and is strongly related to markers of social disadvantage. Finally, Haetzman et al. (2003)[15] using a postal survey in the U.K. reported that 53.8% endorsed having chronic pain. Little additional detail concerning the prevalence of chronic pain was given however since the focus of this study was on the relationship between chronic pain and care-seeking.

Summary

Prolonged pain is common in the general population of adults, with the median estimate approximately 15%.[9] Differences in estimates of prevalence rates for chronic pain do not appear to be systematically related to variations in study methodology or inclusion criteria based on the duration of pain.[9] Increased pain prevalence has been reported in women, older persons and persons with lower income.[9, 12, 14]

Chronic Pain and Use of Conventional Medicine

Despite evidence that chronic pain is a significant problem in the general population, very few studies have examined the association between chronic pain and utilization of health services. Most studies to date have focused on use of conventional medical care including consultations with a general practitioner (GP) or physical therapist, overnight hospital admissions, hospital emergency department (ED) visits. A few studies have also examined self-care practices and use of complementary or alternative medicine (CAM) approaches (discussed below). Notably, these studies have been conducted in a number of different countries, each with their own health care system. Nevertheless, there are areas of consensus in the reported findings as highlighted below.

The earliest study examining the relationship between chronic pain and use of health care was conducted in the U.S. by Von Korff and colleagues (1991)[2] in a probability sample of 1016 adult enrollees in a Health Maintenance Organization (HMO). This study sought to determine whether pain characteristics (e.g., severity, persistence) and psychological distress predicted the likelihood of care-seeking for a painful symptom. The study also sought to examine the overall impact of chronic pain on use of ambulatory health care. Pain was assessed using a questionnaire which asked about pain problems of the back, head, abdomen, chest and temporomandibular region in the prior 6 months. The latter was included to allow comparison with 242 patients with temporomandibular disorder (TMD). The questionnaire assessed the persistence of the pain over the previous 6 months, daily duration of pain, typical intensity of pain, pain-related interference with daily activities and the number of days in the prior 6 months when the respondent was unable to conduct usual activities due to pain. Pain severity was measured by the sum of the ratings for persistence, intensity and interference. Persistent pain was defined as pain being present on more than half the days in the previous 6 months.

Respondents were also asked for each reported pain problem whether they had sought care from a doctor, physical therapist, chiropractor, or other health care professional in the previous 6 months. Dentists were included instead of physical therapists for TMD pain and headaches. Automated data was used to assess total use of ambulatory care by respondents in the year prior to and the year following the survey. Ambulatory care included primary care, specialty care and emergency/walk-in visits.

Multivariate analyses revealed that pain severity and pain persistence were the strongest and most consistent predictors of health care contact for a painful symptom. These findings held after controlling for age, sex, recency of pain onset, self-rated health, and psychological distress. Thus, persons with more persistent and more severe pain symptoms were significantly more likely to seek care for that symptom compared with persons whose pain was nonpersistent or less severe. To illustrate, among respondents with persistent headache, 45% had used health care for headache in the prior 6 months compared to 17% of respondents with nonpersistent headache. Similarly, the likelihood of health care contact rose from 9% for respondents with mild headache to 29% for those with severe headache. Moreover, for headache, the adjusted odds ratio (OR) for a health care contact was 8.2 for severe pain compared to mild pain and 5.8 for persistent pain relative to nonpersistent pain. Poorer self-rated health status was associated with increased care-seeking for headache and abdominal pain, although psychological distress was not associated with increased health care contact. Finally, sex of the respondent was not related to likelihood of care-seeking nor was age clearly associated with the probability of health care contact.

To examine the impact of chronic pain on total ambulatory care, pain status was summarized across the five anatomical sites. Based on severity, persistence and number of activity limitation days, a graded classification of pain status was employed resulting in the following categories (percentage of respondents): 0 - no pain (36.5%), I - non-recurrent pain (18.3%), II – recurrent pain including non-severe persistent pain (37.5%), III – severe and persistent pain with no pain-related activity limitation days (3.6%), IV - severe and persistent pain with 1 to 6 pain-related activity limitation days (1.8%), V - severe and persistent pain with 7+ pain-related activity limitation days (2.7%). Only persons classified as Grade V had rates of ambulatory care in the year after the survey substantially above sex-specific population means (i.e., 4.2 visits per year for men and 5.5 visits per year for women). Thus, Grade V men had 9.9 visits per year and Grade V women had 9.2 visits. A similar association between graded pain status and health care use was found in the year prior to the survey. The same results were found for the TMD cases: only patients with Grade V pain had substantially elevated rates of ambulatory care both in the year before and the year after the survey.

Additional multivariate analyses found that the number of ambulatory care visits in the year prior to the survey was the best predictor of the number of visits in the year after the survey. Notably, after controlling for prior rates of utilization, graded pain status was unrelated to future utilization rates in both the population and TMD samples, although self-rated health status continued to predict likelihood of future health care use.

In sum, the study by Von Korff et al. (1991)[2] found that pain characteristics (severity, persistence) are robust predictors of the likelihood of care-seeking. The fact that sex and age were not clearly related to rates of utilization suggests that increased care-seeking cannot be assumed to be due to sex- or age-related differences in the propensity to seek care, as opposed to differences in symptom prevalence or severity. A relatively small proportion of respondents with severe persistent pain accompanied by significant disability (7 or more days in the past six months) evidenced increased use of health care relative to average rates of utilization. Rates of health care contacts among respondents with recurrent and non-disabling severe-persistent pain were close to the population mean utilization rates. These findings suggest that chronic pain is not uniformly associated with high rates of care-seeking. Moreover, chronic pain status was not related to increased utilization in the year after the survey after adjusting for previous rates of health care use. However, insofar as chronic pain status may have also been a significant factor influencing prior use of health care, it should not be inferred that pain did not influence use of care. Thus, the authors recommend that future research may focus on the role of activity limitation as a possible cause and consequence of frequent utilization of health care.

Chrubasik and colleagues (1998)[12] conducted a postal survey in 1304 adults in Germany which asked if respondents experienced prolonged pain in the previous 6 months. Respondents were asked to specify location, duration, severity and persistence of pain. Information on the number and types of health care professionals that had been consulted, the extent of self-care and satisfaction with each treatment were also assessed. Of the 610 respondents who reported prolonged pain, for 530 (86.9%) the duration was more than 1 year. For pain lasting longer than 1 year, estimated prevalence of mild pain was 11%, severe 25%, and intolerable 3.5%. The most common compliant was musculoskeletal pain from one or more sites, with or without pain complaints that were not musculoskeletal. One third of respondents with prolonged pain reported seeing care from more than one health care professional (HCP): GP's and specialists in physical medicine were the most commonly consulted. Thus, in the total sample that reported pain, 12.3% used self-care or consulted non-HCPs, 48.9% consulted 1 HCP, 24.3% consulted 2 HCPs, 3.9% consulted 3 HCPs and 0.7% consulted more than 3 HCPs.

Multivariate analyses revealed consistent associations between pain severity, pain duration, number of pain sites, number of HCPs consulted, and the number of treatments tried. Additional multivariate analyses revealed that increasing age, increased pain intensity, number of pain sites, and pain duration were identified as independent predictors of the number of health care visits. Overall treatment satisfaction was 75% among those with pain but this fell to 30% in those with persistent and intolerable pain. Multivariate analyses identified older age, number of HCPs consulted, number of pain sites, and pain intensity as predictors of lowered treatment satisfaction.

Thus, in this study, pain characteristics (duration, severity) as well as older age were the main predictors of care-seeking. Chrubasik et al. (1998)[12] noted that their prevalence estimates of 40% for chronic pain in the general population mirrored those of prior studies [11, 13]. The authors therefore point out that the stability of estimated prevalence of chronic pain across nearly a decade is inconsistent with the notion that more effective treatments for pain have become available during this time period.[16] On the other hand, it is also possible that improvements in treatments were offset by increased prevalence of pain in the population due to the overall aging of the population or other unaccounted for demographic changes. However, their findings of low treatment satisfaction among respondents with persistent, intolerable pain suggest that despite increased consumption of health care, these patients have been unsuccessful in their quest for adequate pain management.

Andersson and colleagues (1999)[17] conducted a postal survey on chronic pain and use of health care in the general adult population in Sweden. Chronic pain was defined as recurrent or persistent pain lasting for more than 3 months. Health care utilization was estimated from items assessing number of visits to physicians, physical therapists and CAM practitioners (the latter are discussed below) in the past 3 months. Primary care providers (PCPs) were the most frequently consulted HCPs by respondents with pain. Thus, 39.5% of respondents reporting chronic pain had visited a PCP compared to 25.5% of those without pain, after controlling for age ($p < .05$). However, there were no sex differences in number of PCP visits (2.7 for men; 2.8 for women). Respondents with shorter pain duration (3-6 months) had more visits (59%) than those with longer pain duration (> 6 months; 34%). In addition, more chronic pain respondents (7.2%) reported at least one visit to a physical therapist compared to those without chronic pain (1.2%) but there were no sex differences in the number of these visits.

When respondents reporting high pain intensity (grade 4-5) were examined, those with depression, insomnia, nervousness and widespread pain were significantly more likely to see a PCP than those without these characteristics. Care seekers were more likely to have taken at least 1 sick day in the past 3 months and to have used analgesics (both with and without a prescription). Multivariate analyses in respondents with chronic pain showed that white collar workers were more likely than blue collar workers to consult a PCP and immigrants more likely than non-immigrants to seek such care. High pain intensity, depressive symptoms and older age predicted increased care-seeking after controlling for SES, ethnicity (immigrant status), self-care activities, and diagnosis with chronic disease. Comparable analyses in respondents without chronic pain indicated that depressive symptoms and presence of chronic disease were the only predictors of increased likelihood of care-seeking.

Thus, the findings of Andersson et al. (1999)[17] indicated that traditional consultations with PCPs and physical therapists were more common in respondents with chronic pain than those without chronic pain. However, there were no differences in hospitalizations between respondents with and without chronic pain. Notably, in contrast to the earlier studies by Von Korff et al. (1991)[2] and Chrubasik et al. (1998)[12], this study did not ask respondents to specify whether they sought care specifically for pain. Instead, overall health care use was assessed. Nevertheless, Andersson et al. concluded that the utilization of health care among individuals with chronic pain depends primarily on perceptions of pain intensity, independent of pain location, but is also influenced by ethnicity (including immigration status) age, socioeconomic status (SES) and depression symptoms.

Haetzman and colleagues (2003)[15] assessed use of conventional and alternative therapy by individuals who reported chronic pain with a mailed survey conducted in the U. K. In this study, health care utilization was evaluated only among individuals with chronic pain (i.e., lasting 3 months or more) and there were no comparisons with rates of utilization in non-chronic pain respondents. The survey assessed how often respondents with chronic pain visited a GP, hospital specialist, physical therapist, or an alternative practitioner in the prior year (the latter is discussed below). Results indicated that the GP was the most frequently consulted HCP, with 67.2% of respondents reporting having visited their GP in the previous 12 months. There were no sex differences but older individuals consulted the GP more often than younger individuals. Hospital specialists were visited by 34% of respondents, and physical therapists were consulted by 25.9% of respondents. Increased pain severity was associated with increased likelihood of consulting GPs, hospital specialists, and physical therapists, as well as alternative therapists (discussed below).

The most recent study by Blyth and colleagues (2004)[18] examined chronic pain and use of health care in Australia using a telephone survey. They sought to examine health care use according to chronic pain status in three settings: general practitioner (GP) consultations, emergency departments (EDs) and overnight hospitalizations within the framework of the Behavioral Model of Health Services Use. Chronic pain was defined as pain experienced for 3 months or more in the 6 months prior to the survey; pain-related interference in daily activities was also assessed. Pain status was categorized as: 1) chronic pain with or without pain-related interference, 2) chronic pain with any degree of pain-related interference, 3) chronic pain with: a) no interference, b) little or moderate interference, c) quite a lot or extreme interference. To assess health care use, respondents were asked about visits to the three settings of interest over the past 12 months. These questions asked about use of health care generally and were not specifically related to use of services for pain.

Results indicated that the mean number of health care contacts across all three settings was higher in respondents with pain (with or without interference) and increased with rising levels of pain-related interference. Compared to respondents without pain, the number of health care contacts was between 1.5 and 5 times higher in respondents with the most pain-related interference. In multivariate analyses, having chronic pain with the highest level of interference was associated with an approximate 2-fold increase in the number of GP visits and overnight hospitalizations, and with a 5-fold increase in the number of ED visits, after controlling for age, sex, self-rated health status, comorbidities (history of hypertension, diabetes or asthma), psychological distress and access to care (geographic location and private health insurance).

Although this study by Blyth et al. (2004)[18] did not assess the specific reasons why respondents sought health care, the results are nevertheless consistent with prior work showing that within the framework of the Andersen Behavioral Model, need factors have emerged as having the largest influence.[19, 20] The findings by Blyth et al. confirm that chronic pain is associated with increased use of a range of health services and is directly related to the degree of pain-related disability, which acts independently of other variables. The authors conclude that there is a large segment of the population with chronic pain at potential risk of developing higher levels of pain-related disability which is strongly associated with greater consumption of health care. These findings point to the need for interventions to better manage pain in order to prevent the development of disability.

Summary

Existing studies indicate that in the general adult population, pain characteristics (e.g., duration, severity) are associated with utilization of conventional health services. In those studies which included measures of pain-related disability, it appears that interference due to pain constitutes an independent, robust predictor of health care use. After controlling for pain, the influence of demographic characteristics in care-seeking was less clear. Despite higher prevalence of chronic pain, women did not seek disproportionately more care compared to men. Although older persons have a higher prevalence of chronic pain, at least one study showed no age-related effects on use of health services.[2]

Chronic Pain and Use of CAM in the General Population

The complex nature of chronic pain requires a multidisciplinary approach to assessment and treatment. Thus, this holistic approach may involve use of CAM therapies in addition to conventional medical approaches. According to a recent U.S. study in a representative sample of adults, a high proportion of those who visited a CAM practitioner have chronic pain.[21] CAM therapies have often been used in conjunction with conventional medical treatments, rather than as a substitute.[22-24]. However, only a few studies have examined the use of CAM in adults with chronic pain. One study that investigated CAM use in persons living with HIV is discussed in the section on Special Populations below.

In their seminal article on CAM use, Eisenberg and colleagues (1993)[25] interviewed a national sample of U.S. residents 18 and older in 1991. The frequency of CAM use was highest for back problems (36%), anxiety (28%), headaches (27%), chronic pain (26%), and cancer or tumors (24%). If headaches and back problems (which presumably includes back pain), are combined with the existing chronic pain category, it appears that pain problems would be the most common reason for seeking CAM. In their follow-up study, Eisenberg et al. (1998)[26] reported that the highest condition-specific rates of CAM use in a U.S. national sample in 1997 were for neck (57%) and back (47.6%) problems—conditions in which pain is likely to be a significant problem. Notably, rates of CAM for back problems increased from 35.9% in 1990 to the 47.6% in 1997 (neck pain was not assessed in the earlier survey). Moreover, increased rates of CAM use were reported for other painful conditions including arthritis (1990: 17.5% vs. 1997: 26.7%) and headaches (1990: 26.5% vs. 1997: 32.2%) [26]. Astin (1998)[21] reported that 37% of a national U.S. sample reported seeking CAM therapies for chronic pain, making it the most frequently cited health problem for which CAM was sought. In multivariate analyses, having back problems (OR, 2.3; 95% CI, 1.3-3.5) and having chronic pain (OR, 2.0; 95% CI, 1.1-3.5) emerged as significant predictors of CAM in addition to other demographic and attitudinal factors [21]. Bausell et al. (2001)[27], using data from the 1996 Medical Expenditure Panel Survey (MEPS) (N = 16,038) reported that the most frequent precipitating reasons for visiting a CAM provider could be classified into three broad categories: 1) musculoskeletal (e.g., osteoarthritis, back and joint disorders; 2) mental (e.g., mental disorders related to alcohol and substance use, anxiety or affective disorders); and 3) metabolic (e.g., diabetes and endocrine-metabolic-nutritional disorders). Results indicated that individuals suffering from mental, metabolic and musculoskeletal disorders were over 3 times more likely to have visited a CAM practitioner during the previous year than were individuals suffering from all other health conditions. Individuals suffering from 2 of the 3 categories were more than twice as likely to visit a CAM provider compared to those with only 1 of the 3 conditions. There did not appear to be differences between the 3 categories in likelihood of visiting a CAM practitioner.

Most of the above studies, with the exception of Bausell et al. (2001)[27] examined CAM use that included both self-care (e.g., use of high-dose megavitamins) and well as visits to CAM practitioners. In the study by Andersson et al. (1999)[17] which reported on conventional medical visits discussed above, visits to the following CAM practitioners were also assessed: acupuncturist, chiropractor, homeopath, and naturopath. This study found that during the 3 months prior to the survey, 5.9% of respondents with chronic pain reported visiting a CAM practitioner. The majority of visits were for chiropractic care or acupuncture. In respondents without chronic pain, 1.2% reported CAM use. This rate did not differ significantly from that found in respondents with chronic pain. The authors point out that these results could be due to limited access to CAM practitioners in rural districts surveyed. By contrast, access to GPs in the surveyed areas was good and consultation rates were comparable to other similar studies. Multivariate analyses revealed that high pain intensity and use of self-care predicted visits to CAM practitioners, after controlling for age, SES, ethnicity (i.e., immigrant status), depression, and diagnosis of chronic disease.

An important finding of the study by Andersson et al. (1999)[17] was that use of self-care or CAM was not related to lower use of conventional medical services. Respondents who used self-care had more health care contacts of all kinds including use of CAM therapies. These findings suggest that those experiencing chronic pain utilize self-care, conventional medicine and CAM at high rates and do not substitute self-care or CAM for conventional care. However, as mentioned above, this study did not ascertain whether respondents specifically sought care for pain but rather assessed overall health care use in the prior 3 months.

One other study by Haetzman and colleagues (2003) examined the relationship between chronic pain and use of CAM in the general population.[15] Unfortunately, this study did not compare use of CAM in those with and without chronic pain. Nevertheless, Haetzman et al. found that 18.2% of respondents with chronic pain consulted alternative therapists and 15.7% took alternative medicine. These rates of CAM use were much higher than in the study by Anderson et al. (1999) in which 5.9% of chronic pain patients reported seeking care from CAM practitioners.[17] On the other hand, the earlier study assessed CAM use over 3 months rather than 1 year.

Haetzman and colleagues (2003)[15] found that a majority of respondents (67%) who consulted an alternative therapist also consulted conventional practitioners and similarly most respondents who reported taking alternative medicines (85.9%) also took conventional medications. Overall, women and younger respondents sought alternative therapy more frequently than men and older respondents, respectively. Moreover, the percentage of those with chronic pain who consulted both conventional and alternative therapists increased with increased severity of pain. Higher SES also predicted increased consultation with CAM therapists as well as greater use of alternative meds (and less reliance on prescription meds). Higher SES/education has been shown to be associated with increased use of CAM in other studies as well.[21, 27, 28] But, rather than lack of interest in CAM by persons with less education and lower SES, prior work indicates this difference is mainly due to lack of access to CAM.[29] The study by Haetzman did not assess the impact of insurance. Although the UK has universal health care, coverage did not extend to CAM therapies at the time the study was conducted.[15]

Summary

Pain appears to be a common precipitating reason for use of CAM in the general adult population. Few studies have distinguished between CAM approaches that are self-administered, as distinct from visits to CAM practitioners. In the few studies that have specifically examined CAM consultations, increased pain severity,[15, 17] being female, younger, and higher SES[15] were associated with increased care-seeking. Because consultations with CAM practitioners for pain are likely to be influenced by various factors including availability of such practitioners, and insurance reimbursement, future studies should include measures of these important characteristics.

Psychological Distress and Care-Seeking for Chronic Pain

The link between psychological distress and chronic pain has been well-documented. In their review of epidemiologic studies on chronic pain, Verhaak et al (1998)[9] maintained that there were positive relationships between chronic pain and psychological symptoms (e.g., anxiety, depression) in the studies that investigated such associations.[13, 30, 31] However, less is known about the role of psychological factors and use of health services for pain complaints. Only a few studies have included measures of psychological distress when examining the relationship between pain and care-seeking. As reviewed by Von Korff et al (1991)[2], illness behavior theory posits three psychosocial processes that may influence the likelihood of care-seeking for a painful symptom: 1) symptom perception, 2) symptom appraisal, and 3) situational adaptation to illness. Symptoms perceived to be more persistent and severe are more likely to prompt care-seeking than transient, mild symptoms[32] and theorists have suggested that psychological distress may alter symptom perception such that the likelihood of care-seeking is increased.[33-36] Symptom appraisal refers to the meaning associated with bodily sensations. Thus, it has been posited that a psychologically distressed person may be more likely to attribute such sensations to a disease.[37] Leventhal (1986)[38] maintained that symptoms are integrated by a person's cognitive schemata concerning the causes, identity (symptom pattern and diagnostic label), duration and consequences of a bodily sensation. Such schemata modulate response processes such as care-seeking. Regarding situational adaptation, it has been argued that care-seeking occurs when a person is unable to suppress, ignore or conceal symptoms in a way that permits their integration with the person's daily activities and obligations.[39, 40] Psychological distress may increase likelihood of care-seeking if a painful symptom impaired an individual's adaptive capacities.

Thus, illness behavior theory maintains that persons who seek care for a painful symptom should be more distressed that those who do not make contact for a comparable painful symptom. However, evidence supporting this assertion is mixed. Most of the studies examining this hypothesis have been conducted in patients with irritable bowel syndrome (IBS), a syndrome characterized by abdominal pain and disrupted defecation. Some studies have found greater psychological distress in IBS patients compared to untreated persons with

IBS[41, 42] but others have found no differences in psychological distress between IBS patients, untreated persons with IBS and healthy controls.[43] However, it should be noted that in the latter study somatization (diffuse physical symptoms without medical cause) was elevated in IBS patients and nonpatients relative to controls.

In support of illness behavior theory, Andersson et al. (1999)[17] found that individuals with depression, insomnia and general nervousness were more likely to seek primary health care for pain relative to those that did not endorse these symptoms. On the other hand, Von Korff and colleagues (1991)[2] found that psychological distress (i.e., depression and anxiety symptoms) did not increase likelihood of health care use but distressed respondents more likely to report pain in multiple locations. The discrepancy between the Andersson and Von Korff studies may be due to differences in their measures of psychological symptoms. Although both studies used symptom lists to assess psychological distress, the psychometric properties of the measure used in the Von Korff study, the Symptom Checklist Revised (SCL-90R) [44] have received widespread empirical support.

One study that examined the use of health care for low back pain (LBP) in a population-based survey conducted in Belgium[45] found that health beliefs significantly predicted the likelihood of visiting a health care professional (Adjusted OR = 2.86, $p < .001$), even after controlling for LBP frequency. Specifically, the belief that LBP would be a lifelong problem was associated for increased care-seeking. Although this study did not assess psychological distress per se, it is notable that health beliefs demonstrated such a strong relationship with health care use. Future work should examine the relationship between beliefs about pain, psychological distress and utilization of health services. Given the strong association between chronic pain and psychological factors, studies on the role of pain in care-seeking should include validated measures of a range of psychological symptoms, particularly anxiety, depression and somatization.

Summary

Despite evidence supporting the association between chronic pain and psychological distress, the impact of psychological symptoms on use of health care for pain in the general adult population is mixed. Whereas one study found persons with depressive symptoms were more likely to seek care for pain,[17] at least one study found no relationship between psychological distress and the likelihood of care-seeking for pain.[2] Well-established, validated measures of psychological distress, as well as measures of related constructs such as health beliefs should be included in future studies.

Chronic Pain in Children

Epidemologic Findings

In children, very few published studies have reported on the epidemiology of pain complaints that did not focus on a specific pain condition such as headaches. Perquin and colleagues (2000a)[46] conducted a study in the Netherlands using a mailed survey to assess prevalence of pain in a random sample of 1300 children aged 0-3 years and a representative sample of 5336 children aged 4 -18 years (total N = 5424; response rate = 82%) using surveys distributed at school. For children aged 0-7, the survey was completed by the parent, whereas children 8 years and older completed the surveys themselves. Although a majority of respondents reported experiencing pain in the past 3 months (53.7%), a much smaller proportion (25%) reported chronic pain, defined as pain existing recurrently or continuously for more than 3 months. The most commonly reported pains were headache, abdominal pain, and limb pain. More than a quarter of the sample reported more than one pain site, with the combination of headache and abdominal pain being the most frequent (prevalence = 3.5%), especially in older girls.

Chronic pain was most frequently endorsed in children aged 12-15 years and girls reported chronic pain more often than boys in every age group except the youngest (i.e., 0-3 years). Notably, the sex differences were greatest in the age groups 12 – 15 and 16 – 18 years, with a considerable increase in the prevalence of chronic pain in girls between the ages of 12 and 14. These findings suggest that age or puberty-related factors (e.g., onset of menses) may play critical roles in the development of female predominance in chronic pain. As mentioned previously, epidemiologic work in adults has revealed a strong sex difference in the prevalence of chronic pain in adults. The authors of the study state that the high prevalence of chronic pain and multiple pains in adolescents and girls is a matter of concern for the health care system. Little is known, for example about the extent to which the presence of pain in childhood influences the pattern of care-seeking in adulthood.

Campo and colleagues (2002)[47] examined predictors of recurrent pain in children using data derived from the Child Behavior Study (CBS) which included 395 clinicians from 204 practices in 44 States, Puerto Rico and 4 Canadian provinces.[48, 49] The data represented 21,065 ambulatory care visits in children aged 4 – 15 years. Parents of the children completed measures of children's pain, school attendance/performance, psychological distress, and family functioning. Based on parent report, children were categorized as complaining "often" (frequent) or "sometimes/never" (infrequent) about aches or pains. Multivariate analyses indicated that female sex, age, health status (OR = 3.65 for fair/poor health vs. excellent/good), symptoms of anxiety and/or depression, high rates of health service use (see below additional discussion), lower levels of parent education and family support predicted membership in the frequent pain group.[47] One limitation of this study is that there was no time frame specified in the questions used to categorize children as having frequent vs. non-frequent pain.

In the most recent epidemiological study, Roth-Isigkeit and colleagues (2004)[50] used a version of the survey developed by Perquin et al. (2000a)[46] to examine the prevalence of pain in 715 German children and adolescents aged 10-18 years. Respondents completed all measures themselves (i.e., parent reports were not used in this study). The most common pains were headache, abdominal pain, limb pain and back pain. Notably, pain lasting longer than 3 months was reported by 45.5% of the sample with 35.4% reporting pain duration longer than 6 months. Consistent with the findings of Perquin et al. (2000a)[46], older age was associated with higher prevalence of pain. Moreover, sex differences in pain (greater in girls) increased with age, with no significant sex differences in the youngest age group (10-12 years). The authors conclude that the experience of persistent pain in children and adolescents is common and warrants additional study to delineate the natural course, functional implications and prognosis due to childhood pain complaints.

Summary

Estimates of the prevalence of chronic pain in children range from 25% to 45.5%.[46, 50] Older age and being female are associated with increased pain prevalence. In particular, adolescent girls appear to be at increased risk for chronic pain. Future studies should examine the developmental factors that are responsible for these age- and sex-related effects especially in relation to the eventual adult female predominance in chronic pain.

Chronic Pain and Use of Health Services in Children

Only a small number of studies have examined the role of pain in health services utilization in younger populations. In an extension of their epidemiological study on pain in children, Perquin and colleagues (2000b)[51] reported that in the subsample of children with chronic pain, 57% had ever visited a physician and 39% had ever used medication for pain. Multivariate analyses indicated that intensity of pain, earache and age (in this order) significantly predicted physician consultation for pain. Regarding pain intensity, respondents who reported intensity ratings above 50mm on a visual analog scale (VAS) (0 = no pain; 100mm = maximum pain) were nearly twice as likely to consult a physician. Children with earache were found to have consulted a physician twice as often as children with other chronic pain conditions. The authors speculated that parents may perceive earache as a more severe problem (e.g., fear of deafness). However, they also note that earache may not always be a chronic pain condition but rather recurrent acute pain episodes due to infection. Regarding age, children aged 0-3 were taken to the physician more often than children of other age groups. The authors propose that parental anxiety and/or inexperience with young children may be possible explanations for increased care-seeking in this age group. Notably, the only sex difference in physician visits was among children 0-3 years. In this group, parents of boys consulted a physician more often than parents of girls.

Perquin and colleagues (2001)[52] extended these findings by conducting a prospective study in 507 children (aged 0-18) who reported chronic pain using daily pain diaries that were completed for a 3-week period. For respondents aged 0-11 years, the parent completed the diaries whereas respondents 12 years and older completed their own diaries. Respondents were also asked to document their health care utilization for pain in the previous 3 months. The final sample consisted of 254 respondents (248 reported that pain had ceased during the previous 3 months). Notably, the sample consisted of twice as many girls (n = 173) as boys (n = 80). Results indicated that a GP was consulted by 31.1% of respondents and a specialist (mainly a pediatrician) was consulted by 13.9%. After excluding the youngest age group (0-4 years), girls were more likely to use health services for pain than boys (48% vs. 33%). Pain characteristics (from diary data) showed a strong association with use of services. Respondents who sought care had more frequent and intense pain as well as continuous pain more often than those did not seek care. Interference with daily activities as well as school absenteeism was higher among care-seekers compared to those than did not seek care. The authors noted a high rate of hospital admissions in their sample (6.4%) compared with the national average (4.0%). In addition, they pointed to relatively low rates of use for psychosocial care (2.8%) and CAM (4.0%) in their chronic pain sample. Finally, the authors concluded that except for sex, demographic factors appeared to be similar in those that did or did not seek care, suggesting that pain severity plays a more important role in determining health care use. However, it should be noted that one limitation of this study was that it did not use multivariate analyses.

Campo and colleagues (2002)[47] in the study using CBS data cited above examined the relationships among recurrent pain, emotional distress and health care use. Parents provided data on the number of outpatient visits (primary care or emergency room), number of overnight hospital admissions and mental health visits in the previous 6 months. Children who were in the frequent pain group (described above) had significantly more ambulatory medical visits (3.7 vs. 2.2, $p < .001$) and were more likely to have seen a mental health provider than those in the non-frequent pain group. The study also examined health care visits for medically unexplained symptoms. Children whose parents answered "often" or "sometime" to the following question were categorized as having a history of medical visits for unexplained symptoms, "Does this child have a history of visiting the doctor with the doctor finding nothing wrong?" Multivariate analyses indicated that being in the frequent pain group (OR = 2.47) and internalizing psychopathology (anxiety/depression) (OR = 1.91) were significant predictors of medical visits for unexplained symptoms. Finally, predictors of high health care use, defined as > 4 ambulatory visits in the past 6 months, were examined in multivariate analyses. Negative parent perceptions of child health (OR = 4.97), frequent pain (OR = 2.14), internalizing symptoms (OR = 1.32) and lower levels of family support (OR = 1.26) were significant predictors of high health care use.

Campo et al. (2002)[47] conclude that negative parent perceptions of child health were predictive of recurrent pain in their children, as well as medical visits for unexplained symptoms and higher levels of health services use. They maintain that their findings are consistent with prior work showing that parent health beliefs and attention to illness may influence the experience of pain and development of associated impairment.[53] However, one limitation of this study is that it relied completely on parent ratings and did not include children's perceptions of their own pain. Because pain is subjective, it has been noted that self-report of pain should be considered the "gold standard" for pain assessment.[54] Campo et al. also note that the strong relationship between recurrent pain and internalizing psychopathology poses a challenge to the current health care delivery system that often segregates systems of care for mental and physical health. They suggest that integrated models of service delivery are worthy of consideration for children with recurrent pain.

Recently, we examined the relationship between child self-reported pain symptoms and health care utilization in a convenience sample of 225 (111 girls; 49.3%) children aged 8- 18 years (mean = 12.5 years). Children were asked if they had experienced any of a list of pain problems at least once a month, in the past three months. A high proportion (n = 179; 79%) of the sample endorsed at least one pain problem, with the most common being headache, stomachache and pain in the arms/legs. Of those children who reported pain, 31 (17.3%) reported seeing a health care professional for the pain. Older age, frequency of pain and degree of functional impairment were associated with having sought care for pain. Functional impairment due to pain was assessed across the following domains: school work, social activities, physical activities/sport, eating and sleeping. Additional analysis revealed that functional impairment related to physical activities/sport was most strongly associated with seeing a health care professional. There were no differences in sex, race/ethnicity, anxiety, depression or somatization between children who did or did not seek care. Although these findings were derived from a small, convenience sample and the chronicity of pain was not ascertained, it is notable that pain severity and degree of functional impairment emerged as correlates of care-seeking in children. These findings mirror those of Von Korff et al (1991)[2] and Blyth et al (2004)[18] in adults—both of these studies suggested that pain-related disability as well as pain severity were important predictors of health care use. Thus, future studies on care-seeking in children should examine the extent to which functional impairment related to pain contributes to services utilization.

Very few studies have examined child self-initiated health care use since for most pediatric health care visits, parents are involved and are typically the initiators of care-seeking. Although rare, some schools have instituted "open systems" wherein children may seek care without the involvement of parents or teachers. Because such visits are purely child-initiated, they may provide a window on future care-seeking behaviors. Thus, Lewis and Lewis (1989)[55] reported that girls (but not boys) who made frequent self-initiated nurse visits within an open system during a 2 year period at ages 7-12 years, showed a similar pattern of frequent care-seeking at adults 12 years later. These frequent users did not have more medical problems and the most common reasons for visiting the school nurse were headaches and stomachaches. Their findings suggest that being female and making more visits for functional pain complaints as a child are associated with a greater likelihood of increased care-seeking in young adulthood.

Tsao and Zeltzer (2003)[56] examined relationships among sex, pain-related complaints and school nurse visits in 57 children (36 girls) aged 9-11 within an "open system." In this system, "care cards" were place in boxes throughout the school and to see a nurse, the child took a "care card" from a box and went directly to the nurse without seeking permission from school personnel. In this study, children completed a self-report measure of pain-related symptoms and data on nurse visits was collected prospectively over a 1 year period. Multivariate analyses revealed that for girls only, increased pain symptoms predicted more total self-initiated visits and more visits for complaints with documented physical findings (e.g., fever). However, for both boys and girls, greater pain symptoms predicted more visits for complaints *without* documented physical findings (e.g., stomachaches). Total nurse visits were not related to sex or to pain scores. The finding that higher levels of pain report were associated with increased likelihood of self-initiated care in girls held mainly for complaints with documented physical findings, suggestive of early illness, rather than for functional complaints, such as abdominal pain or headaches. One possible explanation is that girls in this sample simply experienced more acute illnesses or noticed symptoms of acute illnesses earlier than boys. Unfortunately, the study did not include measures of actual illness incidence, including students who sought out the nurse and those who did not. While the study did not suggest that girls had a lower threshold for noticing and/or reporting symptoms than boys since there were no sex difference in pain scores, those girls who did report more pain-related symptoms may also have had a lower threshold for seeking care once symptoms were perceived. Thus, this study may have identified the subgroup of girls with heightened attention to pain symptoms and greater willingness to act on them, with both conditions combined perhaps as the precursors to the adult/late adolescent female pattern of increased health-seeking for pain conditions. Overall, the findings in this small convenience sample support the notion that baseline pain symptoms in pre-adolescent children are predictive of self-initiated visits for care, particularly for functional symptoms over a 1 year period.

It should be noted that despite the findings above, at least one study found no relationship between chronic pain in children and the likelihood of consulting a GP.[57] Using the measure developed by Perquin et al. (2000a)[46], van Eekelen and colleagues surveyed a random sample of children aged 0-18 years (n = 1316) from ten general practices in the Netherlands. Based on their responses, children were categorized as having chronic pain (i.e., pain lasting more than 3 months) (n = 95) or as controls (i.e., pain lasting less than 3 months or no pain) (n = 105). Using GPs' medical records, all contacts including home visits, consultations and telephone calls were counted for the year prior to the survey and for a two-year period after the survey. Results indicated that for both groups the average consultation rate during the three year period was 2.6 contacts per year (SD = 2.2, median = 2.0, range = 0 – 13.7), and there were no age or sex differences in consultation rates. Although this study had the advantage of using data drawn from medical records and did assess health care use prospectively, it is unclear whether children's pain status was reviewed at any point after the initial assessment. As noted above in the study by Perquin et al. (2001)[52], in their sample of 507 respondents with chronic pain, 48.9% (n = 248) reported that pain had ceased during the previous 3 months. Thus, it is possible that a proportion of those who were initially classified as belonging in the chronic pain group would have stopped having pain at some point during the study period.

Summary

In children, pain characteristics and pain-related interference have been shown to predict use of health services. One study also found that negative parent perceptions of their child's health was also associated with an increased likelihood of care-seeking.[47] Strong relationships have emerged between psychosocial factors (e.g., internalizing symptoms; school absenteeism) and greater use of health services for pain in children. In the very young (0-4 years), parents of boys were more likely to seek care for pain compared to parents of girls.[51] However, in older age groups, girls were more like to use health care for pain relative to boys.[52]

SPECIAL POPULATIONS

Persons Living with HIV

Researchers have also examined the impact of pain on access to health care among vulnerable populations other than children. For example, a limited number of studies have examined the role of pain in the use of health services among persons living with HIV and AIDS. In recognizing the negative impact of pain on health-related quality of life (HRQOL) for persons with HIV and that pain may be an important factor in seeking medical care, Dobalian et al. (2004)[58] investigated the effect of pain on the use of outpatient services among a nationally representative sample of adults receiving medical care for HIV in the contiguous U.S.. This study used Poisson regression to assess outpatient utilization based on respondents' reports of the number of times they visited an outpatient provider (HMO, private MD, community clinic, hospital clinic, other medical clinic, or usual provider) over a six month period. The sample included 2,267 respondents from the HIV Cost and Services Utilization Study (HCSUS). The study was guided by Andersen's Behavioral Model of Health Services Use. Key predisposing characteristics included sex and race/ethnicity, enabling characteristics included income and insurance, and need characteristics included pain, CD4 count, and diagnosis with AIDS.

To assess pain, the researchers used the pain subscale of the Short Form-36 (SF-36), a widely used and psychometrically sound instrument for measuring the health status of respondents.[59, 60] The scale was derived from the following two questions: 1) "During the past four weeks, how much did pain interfere with your normal work (including work outside the house and housework)? Would you say: not at all (1), a little bit (2), moderately (3), quite a bit (4), or extremely (5)?" and 2) "How much bodily pain have you had during the past four weeks? Would you say: none (1), very mild (2), mild (3), moderate (4), severe (5), or very severe (6)?"

The study noted that 67% of respondents reported experiencing pain during the previous four week period. Self-reported bodily pain was higher among persons with an AIDS diagnosis, women who were exposed to HIV via intravenous (IV) drug use, the unemployed, and those without a baccalaureate degree, but lower among African Americans. The researchers found that patients reporting more pain and those developing more pain between baseline and 6 month follow-up used more outpatient services. Furthermore, poorer health (CD4 count <50 cells/mm^3, less energy as assessed by the vitality subscale of the SF-36) was associated with higher use.

Using the results of the Poisson regression, Dobalian et al. (2004)[58] also modeled predicted values for the number of annual outpatient visits based on varying levels of pain to demonstrate the size of the effect of pain on outpatient use. They found that the predicted difference in the number of visits between those without pain and those with the maximum amount of pain at follow-up was about 4.1 visits annually. The authors concluded that pain is an important need characteristic by itself, regardless of objective clinical health status indicators (CD4 count and diagnosis with AIDS), and noted that change in pain (i.e., increasing pain over time) had a substantial impact on utilization even after controlling for health status. The authors suggested that improved pain management for persons with pain and better detection of persons at risk for developing pain might lead to a reduction in the use of outpatient services and health-related expenditures.

A few other studies have also sought to examine the role of pain in the use of alternative therapies by persons living with HIV and AIDS. Fairfield et al. (1998)[61] found that pain or neuropathy was the most common reason for visiting a CAM provider among a convenience sample of 180 HIV patients (33% of respondents). A study of 256 HIV+ persons reported that pain was associated with CAM use.[62] In contrast, a study that sampled 70 HIV+ gay men found that respondents with little or no pain were more likely to use CAM.[63] However, these studies used relatively small convenience samples, and thus their generalizability was limited, particularly among the poor and racial and ethnic minorities.

Using a nationally representative U.S. sample, Tsao et al. (2005)[64] investigated the relationship of bodily pain to the use of CAM using data from a different wave of the HCUS that included 2,466 adults living with HIV. The researchers conceptualized pain as a need characteristic within the context of the predisposing, enabling, and need characteristics (PEN) of Andersen's Behavioral Model of Health Services Use, and used the same pain subscale from the SF-36 used in Dobalian et al.(2004).[58] Tsao and colleagues used multivariate analyses to examine the association of baseline PEN characteristics with the use of CAM approximately 6 months later, including use of five specific CAM domains based on groupings used by the National Center for Complementary and Alternative Medicine

(NCCAM; http://nccam.nih.gov/health/whatiscam/ website viewed 4/9/05). Change in pain was also examined in relation to CAM use. The five domains and the individual therapies included in each domain were: mind-body interventions (i.e., relaxation, spiritual healing, self-help groups, imagery, biofeedback, and hypnosis), biologically-based therapies (i.e., herbal medicine, megavitamin therapy, underground/unlicensed drugs, and lifestyle diets), manipulative/body-based methods (i.e., massage and chiropractic care), alternative medical systems (i.e., homeopathy, acupuncture, and folk remedies), and energy therapies (i.e., energy healing). The researchers found that pain at baseline was a strong predictor of subsequent CAM use across all domains except energy healing. The researchers noted that the lack of an association between pain and energy healing may have been due to the small number of patients who endorsed its use.

The Tsao et al. (2005)[64] study is also notable in that it included psychological symptoms (e.g., anxiety, depression) as well as substance abuse (i.e., drug dependence, heavy alcohol drinker) as need characteristics. Respondents were classified as having screened positive or negative for an anxiety or depressive disorder during the past year based on the short form of the World Health Organization's Composite International Diagnostic Interview (CIDI-SF).[65] Drug dependence was defined as use without a doctor's prescription, in larger amounts than prescribed, or for a longer period than prescribed, of any of eight classifications of drugs (analgesics, amphetamines, cocaine, hallucinogens, heroin, inhalants, marijuana, sedatives) during the past 12 months, and if the respondent reported using more than intended or having emotional/psychiatric problems related to the use. Heavy alcohol drinkers were defined as those who drank on at least half of the days in the four weeks prior to the baseline interview and who typically had had three or more drinks on those days. The researchers found that depression was an important need characteristic that was independently associated with use of CAM, even after controlling for pain. Patients who screened positive for depression were more likely to use at least one CAM therapy as well as more likely to use mind-body and biologically-based therapies. Finally, depressed patients were also more likely to use a greater number of CAM therapies.

The Tsao et al. (2005)[64] study suggests that pain is an important predictor of use of CAM in persons living with HIV, including both self-care and visits to CAM practitioners. Moreover, patients whose pain declined over time were less likely to have used biologically-based therapies, specifically underground/unlicensed drugs that have the potential to harm the user (e.g., oral interferon-α, disulfiram, and dinitrochlorobenzene). The researchers noted that these findings are consistent with the hypothesis that pain that is poorly controlled may, over time, lead persons living with HIV to seek out untested drug treatments with the potential for adverse effects. Thus, greater efforts at alleviating pain may be directed at HIV populations in order to reduce the use of underground or unproven drug therapies.

Summary

In persons living with HIV, pain appears to predict use of conventional health services and CAM, including both self-care and visits to CAM providers. These associations hold even after controlling for clinical indicators such as CD4 count and diagnosis with AIDS. One study suggested that HIV-positive women with a history of IV-drug use may be at heightened risk for pain,[58] suggesting that persons with a history of substance abuse may be undertreated for pain. Future work should explore the self-medication hypothesis, which in this context, proposes that persons in pain may be abusing substances in order to attempt to alleviate their pain. One study further found that even after controlling for pain, depressive symptoms were independently correlated with use of CAM.[64]

Veterans

Recently, Kerns et al. (2003)[66] reported on pain and use of health services in a convenience sample of 685 veterans in a Veterans Health Administration (VHA) primary care setting. Pain was assessed by asking respondents if they experienced pain on a regular basis and if the pain was a concern to the respondent. Nearly half of the sample (48.4%) screened positive based on their responses to these queries. Data on use of health services was obtained via the VA centralized medical records system for the 12 months preceding the survey, and included the number of: outpatient medical and psychiatric/substance abuse visits, inpatient medical and psychiatric/substance abuse hospitalizations. Medical visits included visits with any medical provider, including visits with associated health professionals targeting patients' medical problems. Use of outpatient medical services was significantly higher among respondents reporting pain (M = 17.54) those who did not report pain (M = 13.4). However, presence of pain was unrelated to inpatient episodes or use of either inpatient or outpatient psychiatric services. In multivariate analyses, age and self-rated health accounted for 5% of the variance in frequency of outpatient medical visits, and presence of pain explained an additional 1.5% of the variance. Despite this relatively modest increment, the authors maintain that their findings support increased efforts to identify and treat those veterans suffering from pain. Even though age was controlled for in their models, it is also conceivable that the overall advanced age of sample (mean age = 65.6 years; SD = 12.3; range = 21 to 91) may have attenuated the relationship between pain and use of health services. Thus, the fact that pain explained a small, yet statistically significant increment in the prediction of health care use in this older cohort is noteworthy.

Conclusion

Ample extant research suggests that pain may be an important factor in seeking medical care. Pain symptoms are commonly experienced in the general population of adults and children, as well as chronically-ill populations including persons living with HIV. Moreover, there is considerable evidence that pain has an adverse impact on health-related quality of life (HRQOL) in these populations. Nevertheless, the relationship between pain and utilization of health services is not well-understood. One significant limitation of much of the literature on pain and use of health care is the paucity of prospective studies. In addition, many studies have not included a broad range of factors that may impact care-seeking, such as measures of pain-related disability, psychological distress and substance use.

A number of studies found more self-reported pain among certain vulnerable populations, including women,[9, 12, 14, 46, 47, 58] and persons who abuse substances.[58, 64] The possible causes of these variations are unclear, but undertreatment of pain symptoms in these groups is one possible explanation. Furthermore, in most studies these groups did not report higher levels of health services use although it is possible that, in addition to undertreatment of pain, other barriers to accessing care may be limiting use of care. Future studies should examine the causes of these disparities, and, based on these studies, interventions should be developed to address this treatment gap and improve quality of care.

The evidence for linking chronic pain and psychosocial problems (e.g., internalizing symptoms and school absences) with health care utilization appears stronger in children. In adults, the evidence for a link between psychological distress, pain and care-seeking seems to be less robust, although larger population-based studies such as HCSUS do provide support for such a link among adults living with HIV. Furthermore, it should be noted that unlike the Von Korff et al. (1991)[2] and Chrubasik et al. (1988)[12] studies, the Blyth et al. (2004)[18] and Andersson et al. (1999)[17] studies were general studies of the use of health services and were not specifically designed to examine the role of pain, which may limit the conclusions that should be drawn from these studies.

Given that current conceptualizations of pain view it as a multidimensional construct incorporating social, psychological/behavioral, and physiological aspects, further study is needed to better understand how these distinct, yet related aspects of pain might interact with other characteristics within the Andersen Behavioral Model in determining health services use. In addition, future investigations should examine whether alleviating pain symptoms leads to reductions in the use of health services. As noted in Kerns et al. (2003),[66] studies of the efficacy of behavioral rehabilitation programs among persons with chronic pain have shown evidence of significant reductions in health care use. [67, 68] This further supports the need for studies examining whether improved palliative care would lead to decreased use of health services. Through improved management of pain, it may be possible to reduce health services utilization among persons experiencing pain and thus decrease health expenditures while also improving the HRQOL of those undergoing care for their pain.

Research in pain and health care utilization has sought to improve our understanding of the factors associated with pain in the general population as well as various sub-populations. By improving our understanding of the characteristics of persons living with chronic pain that predict increased utilization of health care, researchers, clinicians, and policy-makers may be able to better identify the properties of chronic pain that motivate greater care-seeking behavior, develop better systems and processes of care to alleviate those pain symptoms, and improve the HRQOL of persons living with pain, as well as potentially reduce the use of health services and decrease overall health expenditures.

ACKNOWLEDGEMENTS

Research by the first author is supported in part by R03 DA017026-01 (PI: Tsao) awarded by the National Institute on Drug Abuse and by R01 DE12754-01A1 awarded by the National Institute of Dental and Craniofacial Research (PI: Zeltzer). Dr. Dobalian's work is supported by a Veterans Administration Health Services Research and Development Merit Review Entry Program award (MRP 03-328).

References

[1] Merskey, H; Bogduk, N editors. *Classification of chronic pain: description of chronic pain syndromes and definitions of pain terms.* Seattle: IASP Press; 1994.

[2] Von Korff, M; Wagner, EH; Dworkin, SF; Saunders, KW. Chronic pain and use of ambulatory health care. *Psychosom Med*, 1991 53, 61-79.

[3] Koch, H. The management of chronic pain in office-based ambulatory care: National Ambulatory Medical Care Survey. Advance Data for Vital and Health Statistics, no. 123. *DHHS publ. no. (PHS) 86-1250.* Hyattsville, MD: Public Health Service; 1986.

[4] Rosenstock, IM. Historical origins of the Health Belief Model. *Health Education Monograph*, 1974 2, 344.

[5] Phillips, KA; Morrison, KR; Andersen, R; Aday, LA. Understanding the context of healthcare utilization: assessing environmental and provider-related variables in the behavioral model of utilization. *Health Serv Res*, 1998 33, 571-96.

[6] Andersen, RM. *A behavioral model of families' use of health services. Chicago: Center for Administration Studies,* University of Chicago; 1968. Report No.: Research Series no. 25.

[7] Andersen, RM. Revisiting the behavioral model and access to medical care: does it matter? *J Health Soc Behav*, 1995 36, 1-10.

[8] Frolund, F; Frolund, C. Pain in general practice. Pain as a cause of patient-doctor contact. *Scand J Prim Health Care*, 1986 4, 97-100.

[9] Verhaak, PF; Kerssens, JJ; Dekker, J; Sorbi, MJ; Bensing, JM. Prevalence of chronic benign pain disorder among adults: a review of the literature. *Pain*, 1998 77, 231-9.

[10] Kohlmann, T. Schmerzen in der Lubecker Bevolkerung. Ergebnisse einer bevolkerungsepidemiologischen studies. *Der Schmerz*, 1991 5, 208-213.

[11] Brattberg, G; Thorslund, M; Wikman, A. The prevalence of pain in a general population. The results of a postal survey in a county of Sweden. *Pain*, 1989 37, 215-22.

[12] Chrubasik, S; Junck, H; Zappe, HA; Stutzke, O. A survey on pain complaints and health care utilization in a German population sample. *Eur J Anaesthesiol*, 1998 15, 397-408.

[13] Von Korff, M; Dworkin, SF; Le Resche, L; Kruger, A. An epidemiologic comparison of pain complaints. *Pain*, 1988 32, 173-83.

[14] Blyth, FM; March, LM; Brnabic, AJ; Jorm, LR; Williamson, M; Cousins, MJ. Chronic pain in Australia: a prevalence study. *Pain*, 2001 89, 127-34.

[15] Haetzman, M; Elliott, AM; Smith, BH; Hannaford, P; Chambers, WA. Chronic pain and the use of conventional and alternative therapy. *Fam Pract*, 2003 20, 147-54.

[16] Flor, H; Fydrich, T; Turk, DC. Efficacy of multidisciplinary pain treatment centers: a meta-analytic review. *Pain*, 1992 49, 221-30.

[17] Andersson, HI; Ejlertsson, G; Leden, I; Schersten, B. Impact of chronic pain on health care seeking, self care, and medication. Results from a population-based Swedish study. *J Epidemiol Community Health*, 1999 53, 503-9.

[18] Blyth, FM; March, LM; Brnabic, AJ; Cousins, MJ. Chronic pain and frequent use of health care. *Pain*, 2004 111, 51-8.

[19] Korten, AE; Jacomb, PA; Jiao, Z; Christensen, H; Jorm, AF; Henderson, AS; Rodgers, B. Predictors of GP service use: a community survey of an elderly Australian sample. *Aust N Z J Public Health*, 1998 22, 609-15.

[20] McCallum, J; Simons, L; Simons, J; Wilson, J; Sadler, P; Owen, A. Patterns and costs of post-acute care: a longitudinal study of people aged 60 and over in Dubbo. *Aust N Z J Public Health*, 1996 20, 19-26.

[21] Astin, JA. Why patients use alternative medicine: results of a national study. *JAMA*, 1998 279, 1548-1553.

[22] Thomas, KJ; Carr, J; Westlake, L; Williams, BT. Use of non-orthodox and conventional health care in Great Britain. *BMJ*, 1991 302, 207-10.

[23] Muhajarine, N; Neudorf, C; Martin, K. Concurrent consultations with physicians and providers of alternative care: results from a population-based study. *Can J Public Health*, 2000 91, 449-53.

[24] Palinkas, LA; Kabongo, ML. The use of complementary and alternative medicine by primary care patients. A SURF*NET study. *J Fam Pract*, 2000 49, 1121-30.

[25] Eisenberg, DM; Kessler, RC; Foster, C; Norlock, FE; Calkins, DR; Delbanco, TL. Unconventional medicine in the United States: prevalence, costs, and patterns of use. *N Eng J Med*, 1993 328, 246-252.

[26] Eisenberg, DM; Davis, RB; Ettner, SL; Appel, S; Wilkey, S; Van Rompay, M; Kessler, RC. Trends in alternative medicine use in the United States, 1990-1997. *JAMA*, 1998 280, 1569-1575.

[27] Bausell, RB; Lee, W; Berman, BM. Demographic and health-related correlates of visits to complementary and alternative medical providers. *Med Care*, 2001 39, 190-196.

[28] Ni, H; Simile, C; Hardy, AM. Utilization of complementary and alternative medicine by United States adults: results from the 1999 national health interview survey. *Med Care*, 2002 40, 353-358.

[29] Smith, BH; Hopton, JL; Chambers, WA. Chronic pain in primary care. *Fam Pract*, 1999 16, 475-82.

[30] Croft, P; Rigby, AS; Boswell, R; Schollum, J; Silman, A. The prevalence of chronic widespread pain in the general population. *J Rheumatol*, 1993 20, 710-3.

[31] Potter, RG; Jones, JM. The evolution of chronic pain among patients with musculoskeletal problems: a pilot study in primary care. *Br J Gen Pract*, 1992 42, 462-4.

[32] Prohaska, TR; Keller, ML; Leventhal, EA; Leventhal, H. Impact of symptoms and aging attribution on emotions and coping. *Health Psychol*, 1987 6, 495-514.

[33] Katon, W; Kleinman, A; Rosen, G. Depression and somatization: a review. Part I. *Am J Med*, 1982 72, 127-35.

[34] Katon, W; Kleinman, A; Rosen, G. Depression and somatization: a review. Part II. *Am J Med*, 1982 72, 241-7.

[35] Bridges, KW; Goldberg, DP. Somatic presentation of DSM III psychiatric disorders in primary care. *J Psychosom Res*, 1985 29, 563-9.

[36] Barsky, AJ. Palliation and symptomatic relief. *Arch Intern Med*, 1986 146, 905-9.

[37] Mechanic, D. Social psychologic factors affecting the presentation of bodily complaints. *N Engl J Med*, 1972 286, 1132-9.

[38] Leventhal, H. Symptom reporting: A focus on process. In: McHugh S, Vallis TM, editors. *Illness Behavior: A Mulidisciplinary Model*. New York: Plenum Press; 1986.

[39] Alonzo, AA. An illness behavior paradigm: a conceptual exploration of a situational-adaptation perspective. *Soc Sci Med*, 1984 19, 499-510.

[40] Alonzo, AA. An analytic typology of disclaimers, excuses and justifications surrounding illness: a situational approach to health and illness. *Soc Sci Med*, 1985 21, 153-62.

[41] Drossman, DA; McKee, DC; Sandler, RS; Mitchell, CM; Cramer, EM; Lowman, BC; Burger, AL. Psychosocial factors in the irritable bowel syndrome. A multivariate study of patients and nonpatients with irritable bowel syndrome. *Gastroenterology*, 1988 95, 701-8.

[42] Whitehead, WE; Bosmajian, L; Zonderman, AB; Costa, PT, Jr.; Schuster, MM. Symptoms of psychologic distress associated with irritable bowel syndrome. Comparison of community and medical clinic samples. *Gastroenterology*, 1988 95, 709-14.

[43] Welch, GW; Hillman, LC; Pomare, EW. Psychoneurotic symptomatology in the irritable bowel syndrome: a study of reporters and non-reporters. *Br Med J (Clin Res Ed)*, 1985 291, 1382-4.

[44] Derogatis, LR. SCL-90-R Symptom Checklist-90-R. Mineapolis, MN: National Computer Systems, Inc.; 1994.

[45] Szpalski, M; Nordin, M; Skovron, ML; Melot, C; Cukier, D. Health care utilization for low back pain in Belgium. Influence of sociocultural factors and health beliefs. *Spine*, 1995 20, 431-42.

[46] Perquin, CW; Hazebroek-Kampschreur, AA; Hunfeld, JA; Bohnen, AM; van Suijlekom-Smit, LW; Passchier, J; van der Wouden, JC. Pain in children and adolescents: a common experience. *Pain*, 2000 87, 51-8.

[47] Campo, JV; Comer, DM; Jansen-Mcwilliams, L; Gardner, W; Kelleher, KJ. Recurrent pain, emotional distress, and health service use in childhood. *J Pediatr*, 2002 141, 76-83.

[48] Campo, JV; Jansen-McWilliams, L; Comer, DM; Kelleher, KJ. Somatization in pediatric primary care: association with psychopathology, functional impairment, and use of services. *J Am Acad Child Adolesc Psychiatry*, 1999 38, 1093-101.

[49] Kelleher, KJ; Childs, GE; Wasserman, RC; McInerny, TK; Nutting, PA; Gardner, WP. Insurance status and recognition of psychosocial problems. A report from the Pediatric Research in Office Settings and the Ambulatory Sentinel Practice Networks. *Arch Pediatr Adolesc Med*, 1997 151, 1109-15.

[50] Roth-Isigkeit, A; Thyen, U; Raspe, HH; Stoven, H; Schmucker, P. Reports of pain among German children and adolescents: an epidemiological study. *Acta Paediatr*, 2004 93, 258-63.

[51] Perquin, CW; Hazebroek-Kampschreur, AA; Hunfeld, JA; van Suijlekom-Smit, LW; Passchier, J; van der Wouden, JC. Chronic pain among children and adolescents: physician consultation and medication use. *Clin J Pain*, 2000 16, 229-35.

[52] Perquin, CW; Hunfeld, JA; Hazebroek-Kampschreur, AA; van Suijlekom-Smit, LW; Passchier, J; Koes, BW; van der Wouden, JC. Insights in the use of health care services in chronic benign pain in childhood and adolescence. *Pain*, 2001 94, 205-13.

[53] Walker, LS; Zeman, JL. Parental response to child illness behavior. *J Pediatr Psychol*, 1992 17, 49-71.

[54] McGrath, PJ; Beyer, J; Cleeland, C; Eland, J; McGrath, PA; Portenoy, R. American Academy of Pediatrics Report of the Subcommittee on Assessment and Methodologic Issues in the Management of Pain in Childhood Cancer. *Pediatrics*, 1990 86, 814-7.

[55] Lewis, CE; Lewis, MA. Educational outcomes and illness behaviors of participants in a child-initiated care system: a 12-year follow-up study. *Pediatrics*, 1989 84, 845-50.

[56] Tsao, JC; Zeltzer, LK. Sex differences in pain-related complaints and self-initiated school nurse visits among pre-adolescents. *J Pain Symptom Manage*, 2003 25, 472-80.

[57] van Eekelen, FC; Perquin, CW; Hunfeld, JA; Hazebroek-Kampschreur, AA; van Suijlekom-Smit, LW; Koes, BW; Passchier, J; van der Wouden, JC. Comparison between children and adolescents with and without chronic benign pain: consultation rate and pain characteristics. *Br J Gen Pract*, 2002 52, 211-3.

[58] Dobalian, A; Tsao, JCI; Duncan, RP. Pain and the use of outpatient services among persons with HIV: Results from a nationally representative survey. *Med Care*, 2004 42, 129-138.

[59] Hays, RD; Morales, LS. The RAND-36 measure of health-related quality of life. *Ann Med*, 2001 33, 350-7.

[60] Stewart, AL; Ware, JE. Measuring functioning and well-being: the medical outcomes study approach. Durham: Duke University Press; 1992.

[61] Fairfield, KM; Eisenbeg, DM; Davis, RG; Libman, H; Phillips, RS. Patterns of use, expenditures, and perceived efficacy of complementary and alternative therapies in HIV-infected patients. *Arch Intern Med*, 1988 158, 2257-2264.

[62] Ostrow, MJ; Cornelisse, PG; Heath, KV; Craib, KJ; Schechter, MT; O'Shaughnessy, M; Montaner, JS; Hogg, RS. Determinants of complementary therapy use in HIV-infected individuals receiving antiretroviral or anti-opportunistic agents. *J Acquir Immune Defic Syndr Hum Retrovirol*, 1997 15, 115-120.

[63] Knippels, HMA; Weiss, JJ. Use of alternative medicine in a sample of HIV-positive gay men: An exploratory study of prevalence and user characteristics. *AIDS Care*, 2000 12, 435-446.

[64] Tsao, JCI; Dobalian, A; Myers, CD; Zeltzer, LK. Pain and use of complementary and alternative medicine in a national sample of persons living with HIV, *J Pain Symptom Manage*, 2005 30,418-430.

[65] Kessler, R; Andrews, G; Mroczek, D; Ustin, B; Wittchen, H. The World Health Organization Composite International Diagnostic Short-Form (CIDI-SF). Geneva: WHO; 1998.

[66] Kerns, RD; Otis, J; Rosenberg, R; Reid, MC. Veterans' reports of pain and associations with ratings of health, health-risk behaviors, affective distress, and use of the healthcare system. *J Rehabil Res Dev*, 2003 40, 371-9.

[67] Caudill, M; Schnable, R; Zuttermeister, P; Benson, H; Friedman, R. Decreased clinic use by chronic pain patients: response to behavioral medicine intervention. *Clin J Pain*, 1991 7, 305-10.

[68] Simmons, JW; Avant, WS, Jr.; Demski, J; Parisher, D. Determining successful pain clinic treatment through validation of cost effectiveness. *Spine*, 1988 13, 342-4.

In Frontiers in Pain Research
Editor: Alexandre Lucas, pp.27-47

ISBN 1-59454-828-5

Chapter 2

THE AFFECTIVE DIMENSION OF PAIN: A NEUROBIOLOGICAL REVIEW

Yu-Qiu Zhang*
Institute of Neurobiology, Fudan University, Shanghai, China

ABSTRACT

The pain experience includes a sensory-discriminative and an emotional-affective component. The sensory dimension describes the quality, intensity, and spatio-temporal characteristics of the sensation. The affective dimension refers to the unpleasantness or aversion of sensation. The great progress at the genetic, molecular, cellular, and systemic level on the study of the sensory dimension of pain has been made over the past four decades. However, "*to consider only the sensory features of pain, and ignore its motivational and affective properties, is to look at only part of the problem and not even the must important part of that*" [107]. A line of clinic observations indicate that the patients with chronic pain suffer from much more affective disturbance than pain itself. Obviously, physiological arousal and hypervigilance to pain cause negative affect, such as anxiety, anger, worry, aversion, even tendency of suicide, these negative affective states in turn enhance pain sensation. Today, more and more attention has been paid to the study on mechanisms underlying affective dimension of pain. In order to deepen and expand our understanding of the nature of pain, this review summarizes the main progress and recent findings from our laboratory regarding the affective component of pain in neuroanatomy, neurophysiology, and cell biochemistry.

Keywords: Pain emotional affect; Anterior cingulate cortex; cAMP responsive element binding protein

---

* Address: Yu-Qiu Zhang Ph.D. Professor of Neurobiology ; Institute of Neurobiology, Fudan University, 220 Han Dan Road, Shanghai, 200433, China ; Tel: +86-21-55522878 ; Fax: +86-21-55522876 ; Email: yuqiuzhang@fudan.edu.cn

INTRODUCTION

"A young boy touches a hot oven plate. Heat sensors in his palm realize that the temperature exceeds a minimum safely threshold and activate sensory nerves in the hand. Within milliseconds, the information is passed on through the arm and the spinal cord to the brain. The brain interprets the incoming information as pain, registers that the hand is in danger of being burned and orders it to retract. Motor nerves in the spinal cord and the arm then transmit this order to the muscles that contract and pull the hand away from the oven plate. The hand is now safe, but the experience of pain caused by the heat remains. The child begins to cry and runs to his mother for consolation. He will remember this painful experience and, on the whole, steer clear of hot oven plates." This story narrated by Professor Herta Flor in EMBO reports [47] vividly depicts the developing of perception, defence, emotion and memory of pain.

The International Association for the Study of Pain proposes that pain is "*an unpleasant sensory and emotional experience associated with actual or potential tissue damage, or described in terms of such damage*" (IASP, 1994). According to this definition, pain experience includes a sensory-discriminative (encoding the nature of the stimulus, i.e. quality, intensity, and location etc.) and an emotional-affective (unpleasantness, or aversion) component. The affective aspect of pain is made up of feeling of unpleasantness tightly coupled to stimulus, also termed primary unpleasantness, and emotions associated with the previous experiences and anticipation of pain, termed secondary affect [121]. The "primary unpleasantness" is the moment-by-moment unpleasantness of pain. The psychophysical experiments have demonstrated that relative to the perceived intensity of the individual stimuli, subjects consistently differentiate among the degrees of unpleasantness evoked by different stimulus modalities. Tonic stimuli (ischemic exercise and cold-pressor) evoke higher estimates of unpleasantness at any given level of pain intensity, suggesting that primary unpleasantness is as much a sensory discrimination as "pain intensity" [122, 126]. Thus it seems reasonable to postulate that the neural circuits mediated primary unpleasantness are at least in part separate from those involved in pain intensity. The "secondary pain affect" is a long-term emotional feeling related primarily to learning/memory, imaging, and cognitive-evaluative factors, representing higher order neural processing [46, 121, 122].

In past four decades, the neuronal structures, pathways, physiology and biochemistry associated with sensory-discriminative component of pain are relatively well established, while the underlying mechanisms of the emotional-affective aspect of pain remain unclear. However, a line of clinic observations indicates that patients with chronic pain in clinic suffer from much more emotional disturbance than pain itself. This review summarizes representation of the emotional-affective aspect of pain, especially secondary pain affect, which will contribute to the prevention and the integrate treatment of intractable chronic pain.

NEUROANATOMY OF PAIN AFFECT

From the peripheral receptor to the cerebral cortex, specialized neural pathways termed the nociceptive system process and nociceptive information. Peripherally, noxious stimuli activate specific receptors (nociceptors) of thinly myelinated Aδ- and unmyelinated C-fibers terminating in the superficial layer of the spinal cord dorsal horn [27]. It remains to be uncovered if subsets of peripheral nociceptors contribute differentially to sensory-discrimination versus emotional-affect. Axons of second-order neurons ascend in the contralateral spinal cord spinothalamic tract to terminate in a number of brainstem sites as well as several thalamus nuclei. Fibers from these brainstem and thalamus nuclei in turn project to the cortex.

Spinal Cord

In the spinal dorsal horn, there are two classes of nociceptive neurons: nociceptive specific (NS) neurons responding specifically to noxious stimuli, and wide dynamic range (WDR) neurons responding to both noxious and innocuous stimuli. NS neurons are mainly located in the superficial dorsal horn (laminae I - II) and laminae VII - VIII, whereas WDR neurons are located predominantly in laminae IV-V [29, 60]. On the basis of the capacity of WDR neurons to precisely encode stimulus features of nociceptive stimuli, WDR neurons most probably contribute to the sensory aspect of pain [83]. The NS neurons appear to encode nociceptive stimulus intensity with some degree of precision, thus its activities are more likely to represent affective aspect [123]. The activities of NS neurons in laminae I/II evidently represent the primary unpleasantness of pain, and ones in laminae VII/VIII process the secondary pain affect [135].

Thalamus

There are four major thalamic nuclei that relay nociceptive input from dorsal horn to cortex. They are the ventrobasal complex (VB), which includes the ventroposterolateral (VPL) and ventroposteromedial (VPM) nuclei, ventroposterior inferior nucleus (VPI), the posterior thalamic/posterior intralaminar region (PoT/PIL) [136], i.e., designated the posterior part of ventromedial nucleus (VMpo) in primate [29], and intralaminar thalsmic nuclei, including the central medial (CM), central lateral (CL), parafascicular (Pf), and paracentral (PC) nuclei. Of these, the VB is considered a "specific" somatic relay of lateral pain system, because the nuclei of the complex receive dense and precisely organized input from the deep dorsal horn (IV to VI), and vast majority of laminae IV to VI and VB neurons are WDR [19, 84, 96]. The VMpo and intralaminar nuclei, the "unspecific" somatic relay of medial pain system, receive somatosensory afferents primarily from laminae VII-VIII of the spinal cord and project to the anterior cingulate cortex (ACC) and insular cortex (IC) [28, 129, 144]. It is likely that VB contribute to sensory aspects while intralaminar thalamic nuclei to emotional-affective aspect of pain [135, 161].

Cortex

There are at least four distinct cortical regions that receive nociceptive input from dorsal horn via distinct thalamic relay nuclei. They are the primary (SI) and secondary (SII) somatosensory cortices of the lateral pain system, the anterior cingulated cortex (ACC) and the insular cortex (IC) of the medial pain system [132]. Anatomic studies revealed SI receives nociceptive projections from lateral nuclei, particularly from the VPL [51, 84], whereas nociceptive projections to SII originate predominantly from the VPI [145]. ACC receives afferent inputs mainly from the medial thalamic nuclei (midline and intralaminar nuclei) [87, 92]. IC receives afferents from the PoT/PIL in rodents and VMpo in primates, PB, and the adjacent SII [137]. Traditionally, SI and SII cortexes are considered to be critical for sensory dimension of pain, whereas ACC and IC are more involved in affective emotional component of pain. However, the corticolimbic pathway from SI/SII to posterior parietal cortex areas and to IC, then from IC to amygdala, perirhinal cortex, and hippocampus [49] suggest that SI/SII may have an important role in both pain sensation and pain affective emotion [121, 123].

In addition to the classical spinothalamic projections, the projections from the spinal dorsal horn have also been demonstrated to the medullary reticular formation, the parabrachial nucleus (PB), ventrolateral periaqueductal gray (vlPAG), thalamic nucleus submedius (Sm), hypothalamic nuclei, amygdale, basal forebrain, ventrolateral orbital cortex (VLO) and neocortex [6, 21, 24, 110, 167, 168]. These pathways and structures may also contribute to the emotional aspect of pain and to the interactions between pain and cognitive process.

Neurophysiology of Pain Affect

Involvement of the cortex and subcortical structures in pain processing has been doubted for many decades. Recent years, positron emission tomography (PET), functionally magnetic resonance imaging (fMRI), single-photon emission computed tomography (SPECT), and whole-scalp magnetoencephalography (MEG) studies explicitly implicate the SI, SII, ACC, and IC in pain processing. Noticeably, recent studies revealed that amygdala is another very important candidate involved in pain and emotion.

Anterior Cingulate Cortex and Amygdala

Anterior cingulate cortex is a part of the brain's limbic system. Classically, this region has been related to affect. Electrophysiological studies have showed that ACC neurons in rats, rabbits, and monkeys respond to noxious stimuli [89, 139, 164]. These nociceptive neurons have very large, often whole body receptive fields, suggesting they are unlikely to be involved in the discriminative aspects of sensation. Furthermore, ACC neurons can acquire responses to environmental cues that predict a painful stimulus [87-89]. Functional imaging studies demonstrate activation of the ACC by both noxious stimuli [25, 37, 67, 92, 117, 125, 153] and film- and recall-induced painful emotion [65, 95, 117]. Using hypnotic suggestion in a population of normal human volunteers, Rainville and colleagues [124, 125] alter selectively the unpleasantness of a painful stimulus (47°C water) without changing the perceived intensity of the stimulus; this reduction in perceived unpleasantness correlated with a decrease in noxious stimulus-evoked activity in the ACC but not in the SI. Clinically, surgical ablation of the ACC and surrounding cortical tissue decreases pain-related unpleasantness/dysphoria and the motivation to avoid painful stimuli without affecting the subject's ability to discriminate the intensity or localization of the noxious stimulus [37, 48, 66]. Animal behavioral studies indicated that lesions of ACC produced severe deficits in avoidance conditioning when noxious somatic stimuli were used as unconditioned stimuli [77, 91, 93]. Also, lesions of the ACC impair the acquisition of a classically conditioned bradycardic response to a cue predicting a noxious stimulus [18]. Using formalin-induced conditioned place avoidance (F-CPA, noxious conditioning) and electric foot-shock conditioned place avoidance (S-CPA, fear conditioning) test, our recent study showed that lesions of the ACC markedly reduced F-CPA, but not S-CPA and formalin-induced two phases of nociceptive responses *per se* [50]. Blockade of NMDA receptors in the ACC prevented acquisition of F-CPA [97]. A recent study from Fields's group [76] showed that excitatory amino acid antagonist microinjection into the ACC in rats before nociceptive stimulus robust blocked acquisition of avoidance learning, and intra-ACC of excitatory amino acid during conditioning produced avoidance learning in the absence of a peripheral noxious stimulus. Such results are supported by other studies showing that scopolamine, a cholinergic antagonist, injected into the ACC results in reduction of pain later on [115]. Additionally, following retrieval of F-CPA task, Fos expression in the ACC was significantly increased [98]. Collectedly, these data intensely support the idea that the ACC mediates both pain-induced negative affect and a nociceptive aversive teaching signal.

The amygdala is a forebrain structure composed of several distinct nuclei including the basolateral (BLA) and central (CeA) nuclei, and is thought to be critical component of the neural circuitry essential for emotional affect, such as conditioned fear [104]. Electrophysiological studies demonstrated that noxious stimuli activated the amygdaloid neurons [12]. Functional neuroimaging studies in humans indicated responses in the amygdala to painful stimuli [11, 16]. Lesions or inactivation of the amygdala decrease emotional pain reactions without affecting normal behavior or baseline nociceptive responses [20, 31, 52, 151]. A recent study from Tanimot et al [150] showed that lesion of the BLA or CeA abolished F-CPA, and intraperitoneal injection of acetic acid-induced conditioned place aversion was abolished by lesion of the CeA, but not the BLA. On the other hand, the lesions of the BLA and CeA failed to reduce the formalin- and acetic acid-induced nociceptive behaviors. Consistent to this result, we demonstrated recently that either lesion of the ACC or amygdala reduced F-CPA, without the changes of formalin-induced nociceptive responses [50].

The neural network of the ACC with the amygdala may also contribute to pain affect. Indeed, many ACC neurons directly project to the amygdala [121, 135]. A very recent study from Zhuo group shows that auditory fear memory induced by pairing the ACC stimulation with a tone was blocked by bilateral injection of the NMDA receptor antagonist AP-5 into the amygdala, suggesting that ACC stimulation produces unpleasantness in mice and form fear auditory memory through its interaction with the amygdala [149].

Insular Cortex

Insular cortex is situated immediately medial to SII on the medial surface of the lateral sulcus. Electrophysiological studies in rats and monkeys revealed that over 40% of neurons in IC respond to noxious stimuli [61, 132, 169]. These nociceptive neurons had large receptive fields. Many of the same neurons respond to visceral, baroceptor and osmotic stimuli [61,

169]. Functional mapping studies have shown that IC is activated by noxious stimulation [33, 36, 68, 114, 116, 148, 153]. Psychophysical tests on a human patient with a tumor which compressed the IC and parietal operculum, revealed abnormally high mechanical and thermal pain thresholds on the left hand. After operative removal of the tumor, the patient regained normal sensitivity [55]. Leision IC results in a syndrome of pain asymbolia and apparently reduces appropriate reactions to painful and threatening visual and auditory stimuli but does not influence pain threshold [13, 54]. So far, considerations of the functional importance of the IC in pain processing have to rely mainly on indirect evidence. The widespread connections among the IC, thalamic, amygdala, hippocampus and cortical regions related to sensory modalities and autonomic functions suggest involvement of IC in autonomic reactions to noxious stimuli and in pain-related learning and memory [132].

Somatosensory Cortex (SI-II)

Primary somatosensory cortex (SI) appears to be mainly involved in sensory-discriminative aspects of pain. Electrophysiological studies have demonstrated some SI neurons in rats, and anesthetized or awake monkeys respond to noxious stimuli. The activity of these neurons correlated with duration and intensity of the stimulus as well as with the intensity of stimulus perception [23, 83]. Human functional brain imaging combined with psychophysical assessment have also provided amount of evidence for participation of SI in sensory aspect of pain [8, 25, 30, 36, 68, 120, 125]. However, 80 % SI neurons are WDR, supporting its role in coding unpleasantness of pain [82]. The corticolimbic somatosensory pathway SI – IC – ACC integrates nociceptive input with contextual information and memory to provide cognitive mediation of pain affect. Clinical observations from lesion and brain imaging studies in humans also suggest that SI may be necessary for the recognition of negative emotions in others as well as self-generated negative emotions [2, 32].

Secondary somatosensory cortex has been defined anatomically in the dorsal bank of the lateral sulcus in the parietal operculum of the monkey. This area actually consists of two different regions in primates, with their own representation of the body surface (termed SII and the parietal ventral area) [90]. Only few nociceptive neurons are found in SII. These nociceptive neurons have considerably large bilateral fields and encode stimulus intensity poorly [39, 40, 113]. Several magnetic resonance imaging and positron emission tomography studies have shown activation in SII after nociceptive stimulation [25, 30, 33, 36, 68, 116, 119, 120, 125, 148]. In primates, lesions to SII cause an absence of escape responses to painful temperatures despite preservation of the ability to detect the offset of noxious thermal stimuli [13]. Patients with damage to the parietal operculum have been reported to elevated pain thresholds on the side contralateral to the lesion [54, 55]. Ploner et al., [118] reported that a patient with an ischemic lesion of the left SII not only grossly impaired in localizing a painful laser stimulus delivered on the affected hand, but also was totally unable to recognize the noxious nature of the stimulus even when appropriated terms were presented to him. However, he can perceive an intense unpleasantness and show appropriate motor reactions and avoidance behavior. These results suggest an important role of SII in recognition, learning and memory of painful events.

NEGATIVE AFFECT AND PAIN SENSATION

It seems generally acknowledge that negative affective states influence pain [41, 70, 138]. According to the IASP definition given above, the emotional response to pain should even be considered an essential part of the pain experience. Pain always has a strong negative affective component. Moreover, pain and negative affect (particularly anxiety or fear) seem to share common response patterns [58]. However, theory and data suggest opponent views on the directionality. Melzack and Wall [108] hypothesized that negative affect increases pain by opening the gate at the spinal level, although they did not specify the exact way in which affective processes might operate on descending pathways. Opposite to the view, Bolles and Fanselow postulated the idea that fear and anxiety inhibit pain and, as a consequence, undermines learning and memory about aversive stimuli [15, 43]. According to them, fear and pain are two different motivational systems, fear being related to defensive behavior, and pain leading to recuperative behavior. An aversive stimulus cannot only engage the pain motivational system, but can also act as an unconditioned stimulus (US). A cue (the conditioned stimulus, CS) that predicts the US elicits an expectation of pain and this in turn generates fear. It is then assumed that engagement of this fear motivational system raises pain thresholds through endogenous opioids and brainstem descending systems. This inhibition undermines the pain state of subsequent aversive stimuli, and thereby, reduces their ability to learn and memory. The findings that a CS previously paired with shock suppresses radiant heat-induced tail flick reflex and paw withdrawal, as well as formalin-induced nociceptive behaviors provide further supporting evidence [44, 158]. Moreover, this conditioned inhibition is attenuated by manipulations that reduce conditioned fear [63] and presenting a CS that elicits fear appears to reduce the effectiveness of the US and undermine learning and memory [45]. On the other hand, some researchers proposed that negative affective states enhance pain based on their wording in the human pain literature [4, 127, 133, 160]. Several studies suggest that attentional factors mediate the influence of anxiety or fear on pain in humans [9, 103]. Pain-related anxiety may be expected to lead to an increase in attention to pain, whereas anxiety caused by another object of fear may be expected to distract attention from pain. There is strong evidence that attention toward bodily symptoms increases the perceived intensity of these symptoms [105]. So, the focus of attention might determine the direction of effects of anxiety or anger on pain, attention directed toward pain leading to stronger pain and attention distracted from pain, attenuating pain, for example, wounded soldiers barely noticing their severe wounds while in combat [99, 106].

Apart from negative emotions like anxiety, fear, worry, and angry etc, pain-related beliefs, arousal, hypervigilance, autonomic and muscular reactivity, avoidance behavior may influence the pain perception also.

POSSIBLE CELLULAR AND MOLECULAR MECHANISMS OF PAIN AFFECT

Given pain affective state and image, cognitive evaluation (anticipation of pain) are inseparable, it is inevitable that pain-related negative affect, especially secondary pain affect, linked to learning and memory of pain-related aversion.

The long-term potentiation (LTP) of synaptic strength in hippocampus has been associated with mechanisms of learning and memory. Recent studies show that similar synaptic long-term plasticity also occurs in pain pathways [130]. The discovery of synaptic LTP in nociceptive systems suggests that learning and memory may share some common neuronal mechanisms with tissue injury, inflammation, and concomitant emotional effect [73, 74, 79, 111, 163].

The cAMP-responsive element binding (CREB) protein phosphorylation is thought to initiate transcription of several target proteins to ultimately enhance synaptic efficacy, and is considered critical for induction of NMDA receptor, dependent LTP, and different forms of memory [85, 140, 165]. In *Drosophila*, induction of a CREB repressor transgene was reported to block long-term memory of an olfactory learning task, while expression of a CREB activator isoform enhanced long-term memory [165, 166]. In rats, injection of CREB antisense oligonucleotides into the hippocampus disrupts consolidation of a spatial learning task [59], while similar injections in the amygdala block the consolidation of the memory for conditioned taste aversion [94]. Finally, mutant mice that lack the α and δ isoforms of CREB are impaired in both a late phase of LTP and in long-term memory of certain behavioral tasks [17]. Recent studies support a similar role of CREB in plasticity in the spinal dorsal horn following peripheral inflammation and nerve injury, suggesting that CREB activation may contribute to a pain-related long-term shift [109, 159]. The recent results from our laboratory revealed that pain-related aversion induced high level expression of pCREB in the ACC, using formalin-induced conditioned place avoidance (F-CPA) task, which has been demonstrated to reflect directly pain-related negative affective state [77, 150], combining with pCREB immunohistochemistry and western blots. F-CPA-induced CREB phosphorylation in the ACC was maximal at 30 min, and persisted at high level at 2 hrs. As compared with sham training group and rats that applied noxious stimulation alone, F-CPA evoked phosphorylation level of CREB was much greater in all time point observed (unpublished data). Taken together, it suggests that activation of CREB in the ACC is involved in pain-related emotional affect.

Four major pathways have been implicated to mediate CREB activation, cAMP/PKA-CREB, Ca^{2+}/calmodulin-dependent protein kinase IV (Ca^{2+}/CaM-KIV)-CREB, mitogen-activated protein kinase (MAPK) / ribosomal S6 kinase (Rsk)-CREB, and cAMP/PKA-MAPK-CREB pathways [53, 62, 101, 156]. Impairment of these signaling pathways markedly reduced injury- and inflammation-induced hyperalgesia and CREB activation in the spinal dorsal horn, as well as the different forms of learning and memory-induced LTP and CREB activation in the CA1, amygdala, and ACC [34, 109, 159].

cAMP/PKA-CREB Signaling Pathway

cAMP is an important second messenger, involving different forms of memory [131, 140], and contributing to long-term changes in synaptic transmission known as LTP [79, 112]. cAMP activates cAMP-dependent protein kinase, PKA, then the catalytic subunit of PKA translocates to the nucleus and phosphorylates CREB at Ser 133 [53]. It has been demonstrated the cAMP-related signaling pathways contribute to the behavioral responses to tissue injury and inflammation [5, 147]. Activation of the cAMP pathway in the spinal cord increased responses of spinothalamic tract neurons to pinch but not brushing, which is prevented by pre-treatment with a PKA inhibitor [100]. Blocking of adenylate cyclase or PKA prevents the mechanical hyperalgesia and allodynia produced by intradermal, intramuscular, or intra-articalar injection of capsaicin [38, 141, 142]. Mice that carry a null mutation for the PKA-RIβ exhibited a significant reduction in capsaicin-evoked plasma extravasation and nociceptive behaviors in the second phase of the formalin test [102]. Additionally, the genetic mutants lacking adenylyl cyclase, PKA, or CREB exhibit significant defects in different forms of behavioral learning and memory including emotional memory [1, 17, 162, 165]. So far, nine different isoforms of adenylyl cyclases have been identified. Among them, AC1 and AC8 are the only calmodulin (CaM)-stimulated adenylyl cyclases [162]. They couple NMDA receptor-induced cytosolic Ca^{2+} increases to cAMP signaling pathways [22]. Recent studies revealed that formalin and complete Freund's adjuvant-induced inflammatory responses were markedly reduced or abolished in AC1 and AC8 knockout mice. AC1 and AC8 are highly expressed in the ACC and IC, and contribute to inflammation-induced activation of CREB. Furthermore, theta burst stimulation-induced LTP of synaptic responses in ACC was completely absent in mice lacking both AC1and AC8 [159]. These findings suggested that the cAMP signaling pathways within the ACC, a central region known to encode the unpleasantness of pain, might link to the inflammatory hypersensitive responses and pain-related emotional memory via activating CREB.

Ca2+/CaM-KIV-CREB Signaling Pathway

CaM-Ks are important modulators of synaptic plasticity and behavioral memory [143]. CaM-Ks comprise CaM-KI, CaM-KII, CaM-KIII, CaM-KIV, and CaMK kinase [81]. Of these, CaMKI, CaMKII, and CaMKIV have the capacity to phosphorylate CREB, at least in vitro [81]. CaM-KIV, also called CaMK Gr has emerged as the most important Ca2+-stimulated CREB kinase *in vivo* [7, 64, 101]. CaMKIV-deficant mice showed the decrease in CREB phosphorylation [64, 128]. Introduction of a dominant negative CaMKIV or dominant negative CREB into cultured cerebellar Purkinje neurons resulted in defects in the late phase of long term depression in response to glutamate [3]. CaMKIV-deficient mice also showed decreased potentiation at a later stage of rat hippocampal CA1 LTP [64]. Neural activity causes translocation of CaM from the cytoplasm to the nucleus and subsequent activation of CREB in the nucleus of central neurons [35]. CaM-KIV as a crucial sink traps Ca^{2+}-CaM complexes in neuronal nuclei. The studies of Wei et al. provided a series of new evidence regarding the role of CaM-KIV in neuronal activation of CREB, synaptic potentiation and behavioral memory. Deficiency of CaM-KIV significantly reduced or blocked CREB activation by noxious shock and synaptic potentiation in the ACC, IC, and amygdale, as well as fear memory induced by a noxious shock, but not influenced behavioral responses to acute noxious stimuli or tissue inflammation [86, 159]. Thus, CaM-KIV may be preferentially involved in cognitive memory related to a noxious shock but not in the behavioral responses to tissue injury and inflammation.

MAPK/Rsk-CREB Signaling Pathway

MAPK family consists of extracellular signal-regulated kinase (ERK, including ERK1 and ERK2), p38, Jun N-terminal kinase (JNK), and ERK5. All the family members are activated by different upstream MAPK kinases (MKKs, MEK), which are activated by MKK kinases (MAPKKK, Raf-1 and B-Raf). ERK is the first and the most studied member of the MAPK family. ERK is most likely coupled to CREB phosphorylation via activation of a member of the PP 90 rsk family of S_6 kinases, RsK2, and subsequently activating cAMP response element (CRE)-mediated gene expression [146]. Accumulating evidence implies the involvement of ERK activation in neuronal plasticity, such as learning and memory [146]. Following contextual and cue fear conditioning, a significant increase in ERK activation in trained animals was observed [10]. Administration of SL327 or PD98059, the inhibitors of MEK, blocked various learning and memory, including fear conditioning, spatial learning, conditioned taste aversion etc [10, 14, 131, 134, 157]. It has also become clear that ERK activation is necessary for the induction of LTP, either NMDA receptor-dependent or NMDA receptor-independent, in the CA1, dentate gyrus, amygdalar, and IC 26, 34, 42, 69, 78]. Additionally, ERK were reported to be involved in pain hypersensitivity. Intraplantar injection of capsaicin or complete Freund's adjuvant (CFA) induced remarkable ERK phosphorylation/activation. Phospho ERK (pERK) labeled neurons were found in the medial superficial dorsal horn of the spinal cord on the stimulated side, where primary nociceptive afferents from the hindpaw terminate. The pERK can only be induced by noxious, but not by innocuous stimuli [71]. Intrathecal injection of PD 98059, a MEK inhibitor, blocked the central sensitization-mediated second phase of the painful response to formalin injection [71, 72, 75, 80]. Our recent study found that pain-related aversion induced expression of pERK in the ACC. F-CPA-induced ERK phosphorylation in the ACC peaked at 5 min, and maintained at high level at 30 min, but markedly decreased at 2 hrs. Microinjection of PD 98059 in the ACC significantly inhibited F-CPA and partially blocked subsequent CREB and ERK phosphorylation (unpublished data). Taken together, it is reasonable to infer that ERK activation might be necessary, but not sufficient for the induction of pain-related aversion emotion.

cAMP/PKA-MAPK-CREB Signaling Pathway

This pathway comprises many key events as it connects the activation of cAMP/PKA with the phosporylation of MAPK. Thus, it is likely that this pathway is of great importance for signal transmission during the induction of synaptic plasticity. Stork and colleagues first described this pathway in PC12 phaeochromocytoma cells [155], and then, Grewal et al [56] detected it in cultured hippocampal neurons also. CAMP/PKA activates Rap1, then subsequent B-Raf, which in turn activates MAPK/ERK kinase (MEK)-MAPK-CREB [57]. Rap-1 and B-Raf are members of the superfamilies of Ras- and Raf-related proteins. Rap1 is expressed in many tissues, including all major parts of the nervous system. B-Raf is abundantly expressed in the brain, such as hippocampus. It has been reported that B-Raf expression is specifically upregulated during LTP [152]. In the mice that express dominant negative form of Rap1 in the forebrain, B-Raf activity was decreased, and MAPK phosphorylation in response to cAMP was reduced in hippocampal slices. The mice exhibited a reduction of LTP when theta frequency (5 Hz) or forskolin were used. Moreover, Rap1-mutant mice showed impaired spatial learning in the water maze and deficits in social recognition. Also, B-Raf knockout mice displayed impaired performance in the Morris water maze, contextual conditioning and social recognition [156]. These data indicate that Rap1 and B-Raf play a critical role in the long-term plasticity. Currently, the cAMP/PKA-MAPK pathway has not been demonstrated activate in the brain in vivo yet.

SUMMARY

Pain has a strong emotional-affective dimension, which is made up of primary unpleasantness and secondary affect. A projection from the spinal dorsal horn through the medial/intralaminar thalamic nuclei to the ACC and IC, called medial pain pathways, is proposed to process information relating to pain-related emotion. The ACC is closely related to pain unpleasantness and may subserve the integration of general affect and cognition. The IC has also been proposed to be involved in affective aspects of pain related to learning and memory. The SII cortex seems to have an important role in recognition, learning, and memory of pain. In chronic pain, physiological arousal and hypervigilance to pain can cause negative affect, while negative affect, such as anxiety, angry, worry and aversion of pain can magnify sensitization and hypervigilance. Pain emotion is inevitably involved in synaptic plasticity and learning/memory. The CREB activation is thought to be critical in induction of LTP and different forms of memory. All the cAMP/PKA, CaM-KIV, and MAPK cascades mediate the CREB activation, which might be related to emotional-affective aspect of pain.

ACKNOWLEDGEMENTS

The authors wish to thank Prof. Chiang ZY (University of Toronto) and Dr. Ji RR (Harvard Medical School) for their critical reading of the manuscript. This project was supported by grant from National Institutes of Health International and Cooperative Grant of USA (TW 7180), and National Natural Science Foundation of China (No. 30370471, and 30425022).

REFERENCES

[1] Abel, T; Nguyen, PV; Barad, M; Deuel, TAS; Kandel, ER; Boutchuladze, R. Genetic demonstration of a role for PKA in the late phase of LTP and the hippocampus-based long-term memory. *Cell,* 1997; 88: 615-626.

[2] Adolphs, R; Damasio, H; Tranel, D; Cooper, G; Damasio, AR. A role for somatosensory cortices in the visual recognition of emotion as revealed by three-dimensional lesion mapping. *J Neurosci*, 2000; 20: 2683-2690.

[3] Ahn, NG; Krebs, EG. Evidence for an epidermal growth factor-stimulated protein kinase cascade in Swiss 3T3 cells. Activation of serine peptide kinase activity by myelin basic protein kinases in vitro. *J Biol Chem*, 1990; 265: 11495-11501.

[4] Al Absi, N; Rokke, PD. Can anxiety help us tolerate pain? *Pain*, 1991; 46: 43-51.

[5] Aley, KO; Levine, JD. Role of protein kinase A in the maintenance of inflammatory pain. *J Neurosci*, 1999; 19: 2181-2186.

[6] Almeida, SM; Queiroz-Telles, F; Teive, HA; Ribeiro, CE; Werneck, LC. Central nervous system paracoccidioidomycosis: clinical features and laboratorial findings. *J Infect,* 2004; 48: 193-198.

[7] Anderson, KA; Means, AR. Defective signaling in a subpopulation of CD4(+) T cells in the absence of $Ca^{(2+)}$/calmodulin-dependent protein kinase IV. *Mol Cell Biol*, 2002; 22: 23-29.

[8] Andersson, JL; Lilja, A; Hartvig, P; Langstrom, B; Gordh, T; Handwerker, H; Torebjork, E. Somatotopic organization along the central sulcus, for pain localization in humans, as revealed by positron emission tomography. *Exp Brain Res*, 1997; 117: 192-199.

[9] Arntz, A; Dreessen, L; de Jong, P. The influence of anxiety on pain: Attentional and attributional mediators. *Pain*, 1994; 56: 307-314.

[10] Atkins, CM; Selcher, JC; Petraitis, JJ; Trzaskos, JM; Sweatt, JD. The MAP kinase cascade is required for mammalian associative learning. *Nature Neurosci*, 1998; 1: 602-609.

[11] Becerra, L; Breiter, HC; Wise, R; Gonzalez, RG; Borsook, D. Reward circuitry activation by noxious thermal stimuli. *Neuron*, 2001; 32: 927-946.

[12] Bernard, R; Besson, JM. The spino(trigemino)pontoamygdaloid pathway: electrophysiological evidence for an involvement in pain processes. *J Neurophysiol*, 1990; 63: 473-490.

[13] Berthier, M; Starkstein, S; Leiguarda, R; Asymbolia for pain: a sensory-limbic disconnection syndrome. *Ann Neurol*, 1988; 24: 41-49.

[14] Blum, S; Moore, AN; Adams, F; Dash, PK. A mitogen-activated protein kinase cascade in the CA1/CA2 subfield of the dorsal hippocampus is essential for long-term spatial memory. *J Neurosci*, 1999; 19: 3535-3544.

[15] Bolles, RC; Fanselow, MS. A perceptual-defensive-recuperative model of fear and pain. *Behav Brain Sci*, 1980; 3: 291-301.

[16] Bornhovd, K; Quante, M; Glauche, V; Bromm, B; Weiller, C; Buchel, C. Painful stimuli evoke different stimulus-response functions in the amygdala, prefrontal, insula and somatosensory cortex: a single-trial fMRI study. *Brain,* 2002; 125: 1326-1336.

[17] Bourtchuladze, R; Frenguelli, B; Blendy, J; Cioffi, D; Schutz, G; Silve, AJ. Deficient long-term memory in mice with a targeted mutation of the cAMP-responsive element-binding protein. *Cell,* 1994; 79: 59-68.

[18] Buchanan, SL; Powell, DA. Cingulate damage attenuates conditioned bradycardia. *Neurosci Lett*, 1982; 29: 261-268.

[19] Bushnell, MC; Duncan, GH; Tremblay, N. Thalamic VPM nucleus in the behaving monkey. I. Multimodal and discriminative properties of thermosensitive neurons. J *Neurophysiol*, 1993; 69: 739-752.

[20] Calvino, B; Levesque, G; Besson, JM. Possible involvement of amygdaloid complex in morphine analgesia as studied by electrolytic lesions in rats. *Brain Res*, 1982; 233: 221-226.

[21] Cavdar, S; Onat, F; Aker, R; Schirli, U; San, T; Yananli, HR. The afferent connections of the posterior hypothalamic nucleus in the rat using horseradish peroxidase. *J Anat*, 2001; 198: 463-472.

[22] Chetkovich, DM; Sweatt, JD. NMDA receptor activation increases cyclic AMP in area CA1 of the hippocampus via calcium/calmodulin stimulation of adenylyl cyclase. *J Neurochem*, 1993; 61: 1933-1942.

[23] Chudler, EH; Anton, F; Dubner, R; Kenshalo, DRJr. Responses of nociceptive SI neurons in monkeys and pain sensation in humans elicited by noxious thermal stimulation: effect of interstimulus interval. *J Neurophysiol*, 1990; 63: 559-569.

[24] Cliffer, KD; Burstein, R; Giesler, GJJr. Distributions of spinothalamic, spinohypothalamic, and spinotelencephalic fibers revealed by anterograde transport of PHA-L in rats. *J Neurosci*, 1991; 11: 852-868.

[25] Coghill, RC; Sang, CN; Maisog, JM; Iadarola, MJ. Pain intensity processing within the human brain: a bilateral, distributed mechanism. *J Neurophysiol*, 1999; 82: 1934-1943.

[26] Coogan, AN; O'leary, DM; O'connor, JJ. P42/44 MAP kinase inhibitor PD98059 attenuates multiple forms of synaptic plasticity in rat dentate gyrus in vitro. *J Neurophysiol*, 1999; 81: 103-110.

[27] Craig, AD. How do you feel? Interoception: the sense of the physiological condition of the body. *Nat Rev Neurosci*, 2002; 3: 555-666.

[28] Craig, AD; Bushnell, MC; Zhang, ET; Blomqvist, A. A thalamic nucleus specific for pain and temperature sensation. *Nature,* 1994; 372: 770-773.

[29] Craig, AD; Dostrovsky, JO. Medulla to thalamus. In: Wall PD, Melzack R editors. *Textbook of pain*. New York: Churchill Livingstone; 1999; 183-214.

[30] Craig, AD; Reiman, EM; Evans, A; Bushnell, MC. Functional imaging of an illusion of pain. *Nature*, 1996; 384: 258-260.

[31] Crown, ED; King, TE; Meagher, MW; Grau, JW. Shock-induced hyperalgesia. III. Role of the bed nucleus of the stria terminalis and amygdaloid nuclei. *Behav Neurosci*, 2000; 114: 561-573.

[32] Damasio, AR; Grabowski, TJ; Bechara, A; Damasio, H. Sub-cortical and cortical brain activity during the feeling of self-generated emotions. *Nat Neurosci*, 2000; 10: 1049-1056.

[33] Davis, KD; Kwan, CL; Crawley, AP; Mikulis, DJ. Functional MRI study of thalamic and cortical activations evoked by cutaneous heat, cold, and tactile stimuli. *J Neurophysiol*, 1998; 80: 1533-1546.

[34] Davis, S; Vanhoutte, P; Pages, C; Caboche, J; Laroche, S. The MAPK/ERK cascade targets both Elk-1 and cAMP response element-binding protein to control long-term potentiation-dependent gene expression in the dentate gyrus in vivo. *J Neurosci*, 2000; 20: 4563-4572.

[35] Deisseroth, K; Heist, EK; Tsien, RW. Translocation of calmodulin to the nucleus supports CREB phosphorylation in hippocampal neurons. *Nature,* 1998; 392: 198-202.

[36] Derbyshire, SW; Jones, AK; Gyulai, F; Clark, S; Townsend, D; Firestone, LL. Pain processing during three levels of noxious stimulation produces differential patterns of central activity. *Pain,* 1997; 73: 431-445.

[37] Devinsky, O; Morrell, MJ; Vogt, BA. Contributions of anterior cingulate cortex to behaviour. *Brain*, 1995; 118: 279-306.

[38] Dolan, S; Nolan, A. Biphasic modulation of nociceptive processing by the cycli AMP-portein kinase A signiling pathway in sheep spinal cord. *Neurosci Lett*, 2001; 309: 157-160.

[39] Dong, WK; Salonen, LD; Kawakami, Y; Shiwaku, T; Kaukoranta, EM; Martin, RF. Nociceptive responses of trigminal neurons in SII-7b cortex of awake monkeys. *Brain Res*, 1989; 484: 314-324.

[40] Dong. WK; Chudler, EH; Sugiyama, K; Roberts, VJ; Hayashi, T. Somatosensory, multisensory, and task-related neurons in cortical area 7b (PF) of unanesthetized monkeys. *J Neurophysiol*, 1994; 72: 542-564.

[41] Eccleston, C; Crombez, G. Pain demands attention: A cognitive-affective model of the interruptive function of pain. *Psychol Bull,* 1999; 125: 356-366.

[42] English, JD; Sweatt, JD. Activation of p42 mitogen-activated protein kinase in hippocampal long term potentiation. *J Biol Chem*, 1996; 271: 24329-24332.

[43] Fanselow, MS. Neural organization of the defensive behavior system responsible for fear. *Psychonomic Bull Rev*, 1994; 1: 429-438.

[44] Fanselow, MS; Baackes, MP. Conditioned fear-induced opiate analgesia on the formalin test: evidence for two aversive motivational systems. *Learn Motiv*, 1982; 13: 200-221.

[45] Fanselow, MS; Bolles, RC. Triggering of the endorphin analgesia reaction by a cue previously associated with shock: reversal by naloxone. *Bull Psychonomic Soc*, 1979; 14: 88-90.

[46] Fields, HL. Pain: an unpleasant topic. Pain, 1999; 6 (Sup) S61-S69.

[47] Flor, H. Painful memories. *EMBO reports*, 2002; 3: 288-291.

[48] Foltz, EL; White, LE. Pain "relief by frontal cingulotomy. *J Neurosurg*, 1962; 19: 89-100.

[49] Friedman, DP; Murray, EA; O'Neill, JB; Mishkin, M. Cortical connections of the somatosensory fields of the lateral sulcus of macaques: Evidence for a corticolimbic pathway for touch. *J Comp Neurol*, 1986; 252: 323-347.

[50] Gao, YJ; Ren, WH; Zhang, YQ; Zhao, ZQ. Contributions of the anterior cingulate cortex and amygdala to pain and fear conditioned place avoidance in rats. *Pain*, 2004; 110: 343-353.

[51] Gingold, SI; Greenspan, JD; Apkarian, AV. Anatomic evidence of nociceptive inputs to primary somatosensory cortex: relationship between spinothalamic terminals and thalamocortical cells in squirrel monkeys. *J Comp Neurol*, 1991; 308: 467-490.

[52] Goldstein, LE; Rasmusson, AM; Bunney, BS; Roth, RH. Role of the amygdala in the coordination of behavioral, neuroendocrine, and prefrontal cortical monoamine responses to psychological stress in the rat. *J Neurosci*, 1996; 16: 4787-4798.

[53] Gonzalez, GA; Montminy, MR. Cyclic AMP stimulates somatostatin gene transcription by phosphorylation of CREB at serine 133. *Cell,* 1989; 59: 675-680.

[54] Greenspan, JD; Lee, RR; Lenz, FA. Pain sensitivity alterations as a function of lesion location in the parasylvian cortex. *Pain*, 1999; 81: 273-282.

[55] Greenspan, JD; Winfield, JA. Reversible pain and tactile deficits associated with a cerebral tumor compressing the posterior insula and parietal operculum. *Pain,* 1992; 50: 29-39.

[56] Grewal, SS; Fass, DM; Yao, H; Ellig, CL.;Goodman, RH; Stork, PJ. Calcium and cAMP-responsive element-binding protein function via a Rap1-extracellular signal-regulated kinase pathway. *J Biol Chem*, 2000a; 275: 34433-34441.

[57] Grewal, SS; Horgan, AM; York, RD; Withers, GS; Banker, GA; Stork, PJ. Neuronal calcium activates a Rap1 and B-Raf signaling pathway via the cyclic adenosine monophosphate-dependent protein kinase. *J Biol Chem*, 2000b; 275: 3722-3728.

[58] Gross, RT; Collins, FL. On the relationship between anxiety and pain: A methodological confounding. *Clin Psychol Rev*, 1981; 1: 375-386.

[59] Guzowski, JF; McGaugh, JL. Antisense oligodeoxynucleotide-mediated disruption of hippocampal camp response element binding protein levels impairs consolidation of memory for water maze training. *Proc Natl Acad Sci USA*, 1997; 94: 2693-2698.

[60] Han, ZS; Zhang, ET; Craig, AD. Nociceptive and thermoreceptive lamina I neurons are anatomically distinct. *Nat. Neurosci*, 1998; 1: 218-225.

[61] Hanamori, T; Kunitake, T; Kato, K; Kannan, H. Responses of neurons in the insular cortex to gustatory, visceral, and nociceptive stimuli in rats. *J Neurophysiol*, 1998; 79: 2535-2545.

[62] Hardingham, GE; Amold, FJ; Bading, H. Nuclear calcium signaling controis CREB-mediated gene expression triggered by synaptic activity. *Nat Neurosci*, 2001; 4: 261-267.

[63] Helmstetter, FJ; Bellgowan, PS. Lesions of the amygdala block conditional hypoalgesia on the tail-flick test. *Brain Res*, 1993; 612: 253-257.

[64] Ho, N; Liauw, JA; Blaeser, F; Wei, F; Hanissian, S; Muglia, LM; Wozniak, DF; Nardi, A; Arvin, KL; Holtzman, DM; Linden, DJ; Zhuo, M; Muglia, IJ; Chatila, TA. Impaired synaptic plasticity and cAMP response element-binding protein activation in Ca2+/calmodulin-dependent protein kinase type IV/Gr-defficient mice. *J Neurosci*, 2000; 20: 6459-6472.

[65] Hsieh, JC; Stone-Elander, S; Ingvar, M. Anticipatory coping of pain expressed in the human anterior cingulate cortex: A positron emission tomography study. *Neurosci Lett*, 1999; 262: 61-64.

[66] Hurt, RW; Ballantine, HTJr. Stereotactic anterior cingulate lesions for persistent pain: a report on 68 cases. *Clin Neurosurg*, 1974; 21: 334-351.

[67] Hutchison, WD; Davis, KD; Lozano, AM; Tasker, RR; Dostrovsky, JO. Pain-related neurons in the human cingulate cortex. *Nat Neurosci*, 1999; 2: 403-405.

[68] Iadarola, MJ; Berman, KF; Zeffiro, TA; Byas-Smith, MG; Gracely, RH; Max, MB; Bennett, GJ. Neural activation during acute capsaicin-evoked pain and allodynia assessed with PET. *Brain*, 1998; 121: 931-947.

[69] Impey, S; Smith, DM; Obrietan, K; Donahue, R; Wade, C; Storm, DR. Stimulation of cAMP response element (CRE)-mediated transcription during contextual learning. *Nat Neurosci*,. 1998; 1: 595-601.

[70] Janssen, SA. Negative affect and sensitization to pain. *Scan J Psychol*. 2002; 43: 131-137.

[71] Ji, RR; Baba, H; Brenner, GJ; Woolf, CJ. Nociceptive-specific activation of ERK in spinal neurons contributes to pain hypersensitivity. *Nat Neurosci*,. 1999; 2: 1114-1119.

[72] Ji, RR; Befort, K; Brenner, GJ; Woolf, CJ. ERK MAP kinase activation in superficial spinal cord neurons induces prodynorphin and NK-1 upregulation and contributes to persistent inflammatory pain hypersensitivity. *J Neurosci*,. 2002; 22: 478-485.

[73] Ji, RR; Kohno, T; Woolf, CJ; Moore, KA. Central sensitization and LTP: do pain and memory share similar mechanisms? *Trends Neursci*, 2003; 26: 696-705.

[74] Ji, RR; Strichartz, G. Cell signaling and genesis of neuropathic pain. *Sci STKE*, 2004, 252: re E14.

[75] Ji, RR; Zhang, YQ. The role of MAP kinase cascades in cell signaling, neural plasticity and pain facilitation. *Neurosci Bull*, 2005; 1: 3-9.

[76] Johansen, JP; Fields, HL.Glutamatergic activation of anterior cingulate cortex produces an aversive teaching signal. *Nat Neurosci*, 2004; 7: 398-403.

[77] Johansen, JP; Fields, HL; Manning, BH. The affective component of pain in rodents: Direct evidence for a contribution of the anterior cingulate cortex. *PNAS*, 2001; 98: 8077-8082.

[78] Jones, MW; French, PJ; Bilss, TV; Rosenblum, K. Molecular mechanisms of long-term potentiation in the insular cortex in vivo. *J Neurosci*, 1999; 19: RC36.

[79] Kandel, ER. The molecular biology of memeory storage: a dialogue between genes and synapses. *Science,* 2001; 294: 1030-1036.

[80] Karim, F; Wang, CC; Gereau, RW. Metabotripic glutamate receptor subtypes 1 and 5 are activators of extracellular signal-regulated kinase signaling required for inflammatory pain in mice. *J Neurosci*; 2001; 21: 3771-3779.

[81] Kasahara, J; Fukunaga, K; Miyamoto, E. Activation of calcium/calmodulin-dependent protein kinase IV in long term potentiation in the rat hippocampal CA1 region. *J Biol Chem,* 2001; 276: 24044-24050.

[82] Kenshalo, DR; Iwata, K; Sholas, M; Thomas, DA. Response properties and organization of nociceptive neurons in area 1 of monkey primary somatosensory cortex. *J Neurophysiol*, 2000; 84: 719-729.

[83] Kenshalo, DRJr; Chudler, EH; Anton, F; Dubner, R. SI nociceptive neurons participate in the encoding process by which monkeys perceive the intensity of noxious thermal stimulation. *Brain Res*, 1988; 454: 378-382.

[84] Kenshalo, DRJr; Giesler, GJJr; Leonard, RB; Willis, WD. Responses of neurons in primate ventral posterior lateral nucleus to noxious stimuli. *J Neurophysiol*, 1980; 43: 1594-1614.

[85] Kida, S; Josselyn, SA; Pena, de Ortiz, S; Kogan, JH; Chevere, I; Masushige, S; Silva, AJ. CREB required for the stability of new and reactivated fear memories. *Nature Neurosci*, 2002; 5: 348-355.

[86] Ko, SW; Chatila, T; Zhuo, M. Contribution of CaMKIV to injury and fear-induced ultrasonic vocalizations in adult mice. *Mol Pain*, 2005; inpress.

[87] Koyama, T; Kato, K; Mikami, A. During pain-avoidance neurons activated in the macaque anterior cingulate and caudate. *Neurosci Lett*, 2000; 283: 17-20.

[88] Koyama, T; Kato, K; Tanaka, YZ; Mikami, A. Anterior cingulated activity during pain-avoidance and reward tasks in monkeys. *Neurosci Res*, 2001; 39: 421-430.

[89] Koyama, T; Tanaka, YZ; Mikami, A. Nociceptive neurons in the macaque anterior cingulate activate during anticipation of pain. *NeuroReport*, 1998; 9: 2663-2667.

[90] Krabitzer, I; Clarey, J; Tweedale, R; Elston, G; Calford, M. A redefinition of somatosensory areas in the lateral sulcus of macaque monkeys. *J Neurosci*, 1995; 15: 3821-3839.

[91] Kung, JC; Su, NM; Fan, RJ; Chai, SC; Shu, BC. Contribution of the anterior cingulate cortex to laser-pain conditioning. *Brain Res*, 2003; 970: 58-72.

[92] Kwan, CL; Crawley, AP; Mikulis, DJ; Davis, KD. An fMRI study of the anterior cingulate cortex and surrounding medial wall activations evoked by noxious cutaneous heat and cold stimuli. *Pain*, 2000; 85: 359-374.

[93] LaGraize, SC; LaBuda, CJ; Rutledge, MA; Jackson, RL; Fuchs, PN. Differential effect of anterior cingulate cortex lesion on mechanical hypersensitivity and escape/avoidance behavior in an animal model of neuropathic pain. *Exp Neurol*, 2004; 188: 139-148.

[94] Lamprecht, R; Hazvi, S; Dudal, Y. cAMP response element-binding protein in the amygdala is required for long-but not short-term conditioned taste aversion memory. *J Neurosci*, 1997; 17: 8443-8450.

[95] Lane, RD; Reiman, EM; Axelrod, B; Yun, LS; Holmes, A; Schwartz, GE. Neural correlates of levels of emotional awareness: Evidence of an interaction between emotion and attention in the anterior cingulate cortex. *J Cogn Neurosci*, 1998; 10: 525-535.

[96] Lee, JI; Dougherty, PM; Antezana, D; Lenz, FA. Responses of neurons in the region of human thalamic principal somatic sensory nucleus to mechanical and thermal stimuli graded into the painful range. *J Comp Neurol*, 1999; 410: 541-555.

[97] Lei, LG; Sun, S; Zhao, ZQ; Zhang, YQ. NMDA receptors in the anterior cingulate cortex mediate pain-related aversion. *Exp Neurol*, 2004; 189: 413-421.

[98] Lei, LG; Zhang, YQ; Zhao, ZQ. Pain-related aversion and Fos expression in the central nervous system in rats. *NeuroReport*, 2004; 15: 67-71.

[99] Leventhal, H. I know distraction works even though it doesn't. *Health Psychol*, 1992; 11: 208-209.

[100] Lin, Q; Wu, J; Willis, WD. Effects of protein kinase A activation on the responses of primate spinothalamic tract neurons to mechanical stimuli. *J Neurophysiol*, 2002; 88: 214-221.

[101] Lonze, BE; Ginty, DD. Function and regulation of CREB family transcription factors in the nervous system. *Neuron*, 2002; 35: 605-623.

[102] Malmberg, AB; Brandon, EP; Idzerda, RL; Liu, H; McKnight, GS; Basbaum, AI. Diminished inflammation and nociceptive pain with preservation of neuropathic pain in mice with a targeted mutation of the type I regulatory subunit of cAMP dependent protein kinase. *J Neurosci*, 1997; 17: 7462-7470.

[103] Malow, RM. The effects of induced anxiety on pain perception: A signal detection analysis. *Pain*, 1981; 11: 379-405.

[104] Maren, S; Fanselow, MS. The amygdala and fear conditioning: has the nut been cracked? *Neuron*, 1996; 16: 237-240.

[105] McCaul, KD; Malott, JM. Distraction and coping with pain. *Psychol Bull*, 1984; 95: 516-533.

[106] McCaul, KD; Monson, N; Maki, RH. Does distraction reduce pan-produced distress among college students? *Health Psychol*, 1992; 11: 210-217.

[107] Melzack, R; Casey, KL. Sensory, motivational, and central control determinants of pain. In: Kenshalo D editor. *The skin sense*, Springfield: Thomas; 1968; 423-439.

[108] Melzack, R; Wall, PD. *The challenge of pain*. Harmondsworth: Penguin Books. 1982.

[109] Miletic, G; Pankratz, MT; Miletic, V. Increases in the phosphorylation of cyclic AMP response element binding protein (CREB) and decreases in the content of calcineurin accompany thermal hyperagesia following chronic constriction injury in rats. *Pain*, 2002; 99: 493-500.

[110] Mouton, LJ; Holstege, G. Segmental and laminar organization of the spinal neurons projecting to the periaqueductal gray (PAG) in the cat suggests the existence of at least five separate clusters of spino-PAG neurons. *J Comp Neurol*, 2000; 428-410.

[111] Nestier, EJ. Molecular basis of long-term plasticity underlying addiction. *Nat Rev Neurosci,* 2001; 2: 119-128.

[112] Nicoll, RA; Malenka, RC. Contrasting properties of two forms of long-term potentiation in the hippocampus. *Nature*, 1995; 377: 115-118.

[113] Ohara, PT; Vit, JP; Jasmin, L. Cortical modulation of pain. *Cell Mol Life Sci*, 2005; 62: 44-52.

[114] Olausson, H; Ha, B; Duncan, GH; Morin, C; Ptito, A; Ptito, M; Marchand, S; Busshnell, MC. Cortical activation by tactile and painful stimuli in hemispherectomized patients. *Brain*, 2001; 124: 916-927.

[115] Ortega-Legaspi, JM; Lopez-Avila, A; Coffeen, U; del Angel, R; Pellicer, F. Scopolamine into the anterior cingulate cortex diminishes nociception in a neuropathic pain model in the rat: an interruption of "nociception-related memory acquisition"? *Eur J Pain*, 2003; 7: 425-429.

[116] Peyron, R; Laurent, B; Garcia-Larrea, L. Functional imaging of brain responses to pain. A review and meta-analysis. *Neurophysiol Clin*, 2000; 30: 263-288.

[117] Ploghaus, A; Tracey, I; Gati, JS; Clare, S; Menon, RS; Mattews, PM; Rawins, JN. Dissociating pain from its anticipation in the human brain. *Science*, 1999; 284: 1979-1981.

[118] Ploner, M; Freund, HJ; Schnitzler, A. Pain affect without pain sensation in a patient with a postcentral lesion. *Pain*, 1999a; 81: 211-214.

[119] Ploner, M; Schmitz, F; Freund, HJ; Schnitzier, A. Parallel activation of primary and secondary somatosensory cortices in human pain processing. *J Neurophysiol*, 1999b; 81: 211-214.

[120] Ploner, M; Schmitz, F; Freund, HJ; Schnitzler, A. Differential organization of touch and pain in human primary somatosensory cortex. *J Neurophysiol*, 2000; 83: 1770-1776.

[121] Price, DD. Psychological and neural mechanisms of the affective dimension of pain. *Science,* 2000; 288: 1769-1772.

[122] Price, DD; Harkins, SW. The combined use of visual analogue scales and experimental pain in proving standardized assessment of clinical pain. *Clin J Pain*, 1987; 3: 1-8.

[123] Price, DD; Verne, GN. Does the spinothalamic tract to ventroposterior lateral thalamus and somatosensory cortex have roles in both pain sensation and pain-related emotions. *J Pain*, 2002; 3: 105-108.

[124] Rainville, P; Carrier, B; Hofbauer, RK; Bushnell, MC; Duncan, GH. Dissociation of pain sensory and affective dimensions using hypnotic modulation. *Pain*, 1999; 82: 159-171.

[125] Rainville, P; Duncan, GH; Price, DD; Carrier, B; Bushnell, MC. Pain affect encoded in human anterior cingulate but not somatosensory cortex. *Science,* 1997; 277: 968-971.

[126] Rainville, P; Feine, JS; Bushnell, MC; Duncan, GH. A psychophysical comparison of sensory and affective responses to four modalities of experimental pain. *Somatosens Motor Res*, 1992; 9: 265-277.

[127] Rhudy, JL; Meagher, MW. Fear and anxiety: devergent effects on thermal pain thresholds in humans. *Pain*, 2000; 84: 65-75.

[128] Ribar, TJ; Rodriguiz, RM; Khiroug, L; Wetsel, WC; Augustine, GJ; Means, AR. Cerebellar defects in Ca2+/caimodulin kinase IV-deficient mice. *J Neurosci*, 2000; 20: RC107.

[129] Royce, G; Bromley, S; Gracco, C. Subcortical projections to the centromedian and parafascicular thalamic nuclei in the cat. *J Comp Neurol*, 1991; 306: 129-155.

[130] Sandkühler, J. Learning and memory in pain pathways. *Pain*, 2000; 88: 113-118.

[131] Schafe, GE; Nadel, NK; Sullivan, GM; Harris, A; LeDoux, JE. Memory consolidation for contextual and auditory fear conditioning is dependent on protein synthesis, PKA and MAP kinase. *Learn Mem*, 1999; 6: 97-110.

[132] Schnitzler, A; Ploner, M. Neurophysiology and functional neuroanatomy of pain perception. *J Clin Neurophysiol*, 2000; 17: 592-603.

[133] Schumacher, R; Velden, M. Anxiety, pain experience, and pain report: a signal detection study. *Percept Mot Skills*, 1984; 58: 339-349.

[134] Selcher, J; Atkins, CM; Trzaskos, JM; Paylor, R; Sweatt, JD. A necessity for MAP kinase activation in mammalian spatial learning. *Learn Mem*, 1999; 6: 478-490.

[135] Sewards, TV; Sewards, M. Separate, parallel sensory and hedonic pathways in the mammalian somatosensory system. *Brain Res Bull*, 2002; 58: 243-260.

[136] Shi, C; Davis, M. Pain pathways involved in fear conditioning measured with fear-potentiated startle: lesion studies. *J Neurosci*, 1999; 19: 420-430.

[137] Shi, CJ; Cassell, MD. Cascade projections from somatosensory cortex to the rat basolateral amygdala via the parietal insular cortex. *J Comp Neurol*, 1998; 399: 469-491.

[138] Sieve, AN; King, TE; Ferguson, AR; Grau, JW; Meagher, MW. Pain and negative affect: evidence the inverse benzodiazepine agonist DMCM inhibits pain and learning in rats. *Psychopharmacol*, 2001; 153: 180-190.

[139] Sikes, RW; Vogt, BA. Nociceptive neurons in area 24 of rabbit cingulate cortex. *J neurophysiol,* 1992; 68: 1720-1732.

[140] Silva, AJ; Kogan, JH; Frankland, PW; Kida, S. CREB and memory. *Annu Rev Neurosci*, 1998; 21: 127-148.

[141] Sluka, KA. Stimulation of deep somatic tissue with capsaicin produces long-lasting mechanical allodynia and heat hypoalgesia that depend on early activation of the cAMP pathway. *J Neurosci*, 2002; 22: 5687-5693.

[142] Sluka, KA; Willis, WD. The effects of G-protein and protein kinase inhibitors on the behavioral responses of rats to intradermal injection of capsaicin. *Pain*, 1997; 71: 165-178.

[143] Sodering, TR.. Cam-kinase: modulator of synaptic plasticity. *Curr Opin Neurobiol*, 2000; 10: 375-380.

[144] Stevens, RT; Hodge, CJJr; Apkarian, AV. Medial, intralaminar, and lateral terminations of lumbar spinothalamic tract neurons: A fluorescent double-label study. *Somatosens Mot Res*, 1989; 6: 285-308.

[145] Stevens, RT; London, SM; Apkarian, AV. Spinothalamocortical projections to the secondary somatosensory cortex (SII) in squirrel monkey. *Brain Res*, 1993; 631: 241-246.

[146] Sweatt, JD. The neuronal MAP kinase cascade: a biochemical signal integration system subserving synaptic plasticity and memory. *J Neurochem*, 2001; 76: 1-10.

[147] Taiwo, YO; Levine, JD. Further confirmation of the role of adenyl cyclase and of cAMP-dependent protein kinase in primary afferent hyperalgesia. *Neuroscience,* 1991; 44: 131-135.

[148] Talbot, JD; Marrett, S; Evans, AC; Meyer, E; Bushnell, MC; Duncan, GH. Multiple representations of pain in human cerebral cortex. *Science*, 1991; 251: 1355-1358.

[149] Tang, J; Ko, S; Ding, HK; Qiu, CS; Calejesan, AA; Zhuo, M. Pavlovian fear memory induced by activation in the anterior cingulate cortex. *Molecular Pain*, 2005; 1: 6-21.

[150] Tanimoto, S; Nakagawa, T; Yamauchi, Y; Minami, M; Satoh, M. Differential contributions of the basolateral and central nuclei of the amygdala in the negative affective component of chemical somatic and visceral pains in rats. *Eur J Neurosci*, 2003; 18: 2343-2350.

[151] Tershner, SA; Helmstetter, FJ. Antinociception produced by mu opioid receptor activation in the amygdala is partly dependent on activation of mu opioid and neurotensin receptors in the ventral periaqueductal gray. Brain Res, 2000; 865: 17-26.

[152] Thomas, KL; Laroche, S; Errington, ML; Bliss, TV; Hunt, SP. Spatial and temporal changes in signal transduction pathways during LTP. *Neuron,* 1994; 13: 737-745.

[153] Tolle, TR; Kaufmann, T; Siessmeier, T; Lautenbacher, S; Berthele, A; Munz, F; Zieglgansberger, W; Willoch, F; Schwaiger, M; Conrad, B; Bartenstein, P. Region-specific encoding of sensory and affective components of pain in the human brain: a positron emission tomography tomography correlation analysis. *Ann Neurol*, 1999; 45: 40-47.

[154] Vogt, BA; Pandya, DN; Rosene, DL. Cingulate cortex of the rhesus monkey: I. Cytoarchitecture and thalamic afferents. *J Comp Neurol*, 1987; 262: 256-270.

[155] Vossler, MR; Yao, H; York, RD; Pan, MG; Rim, CS; Stork, PJ. cAMP activates MAP kinase and Elk-1 through a B-Raf- and Rap1-dependent pathway. *Cell,* 1997; 89: 73-82.

[156] Waltereit, R; Weller, M. Signaling from cAMP/PKA to MAPK and synaptic plasticity. *Mol Neurobiol*, 2003; 27: 99-106.

[157] Walz, R; Roesler, R; Quevedo, J; Rockenbach, IC; Amaral, OB; Vianna, MR; Lenz, G; Medina, JH; Izquierdo, I. Dose-dependent impairment of inhibitory avoidance retention in rats by immediate post-training infusion of a mitogen-activated protein kinase inhibitor into cortical structures. *Behav Brain Res*, 1999; 105: 219-223.

[158] Watkins, LR; Cobelli, DA; Mayer, DJ. Classical conditioning of front paw and hind paw footshock induced analgesia (FSIA): Noloxone reversibility and descending pathways. *Brain Res*, 1982; 243: 119-132.

[159] Wei, F; Qiu, CS; Kim, SJ; Muglia, L; Maas, JrJW; Pineda, VV; Xu, HM; Chen, ZF; Storm, DR; Muglia, LJ;. Zhuo, M. Genetic elimination of behavioral sensitization in mice lacking calmodulin-stimulated adenylyl cyclases. Neuron, 2002; 36: 713-726.

[160] Weisenberg, M; Aviram, O; Wolf, Y; Raphaeli, N. Relevant and irrelevant anxiety in the reaction to pain. *Pain*, 1984; 20: 371-383.

[161] Willis, WD; Westlund, KN. Neuroanatomy of the pain system and of the pathways that modulate pain. *J Clin Neurophysiol*, 1997; 14: 2-31.

[162] Wong, ST; Athos, J; Figueros, XA; Pineda, VV; Schaefer, ML; Chavkin, CC; Muglia, LJ; Storm, DR. Calcium-stimulated adenylyl cyclase activity is critical for hippocampus-dependent long-term memory and late phase LTP. *Neuron,* 1999; 23: 787-798.

[163] Woolf, CJ; Salter, MW. Neuronal plasticity: increasing the gain in pain. *Science,* 2000; 288: 1765-1768.

[164] Yamamura, H; Iwata, K; Tsuboi, Y; Toda, K; Kitajima, K; Shimizu, N; Nomura, H; Hibiya, J; Fujta, S; Sumino, R. Morphological and electrophysiological properties of ACCx nociceptive neurons in rats. *Brain Res*, 1996; 735: 83-92.

[165] Yin, JC; DelVecchio, M; Zhou, H; Quinn, WG; Tully, T. CREB as a memory modulator: Induced expression of a dCREB2 activator isoform enhances long-term memory in Drosphila. *Cell,* 1995; 81: 107-115.

[166] Yin, JC; Wallach, JS; DelVecchio, M; Wilder, EL; Zhou, H; Quinn, WG; Tully, T. Induction of a dominant negative CREB transgene specifically blocks long-term memory in Drosophila. *Cell*, 1994; 79: 49-58.

[167] Zhang, YQ; Tang, JS; Yuan, B; Jia, H. Inhibitory effects of electrical stimulation of thalamic nucleus submedius on the nociceptive responses of spinal dorsal horn neurons in the rat. *Brain Res*, 1996; 737: 16-24.

[168] Zhang,YQ; Tang, JS; Yuan, B; Jia, H. Inhibitory effects of electrical evoked activation of ventrolateral orbital cortex on the tail flick reflex are mediated by periaqueductal gray in rats. *Pain,* 1997; 72: 127-135.

[169] Zhang, ZH; Dougherty, PM. Oppenheimer S.M. Monkey insular cortex neurons respond to baroreceptive and somatosensory convergent inputs. *Neuroscience,* 1999; 94: 351-360.

In Frontiers in Pain Research
Editor: Alexendre Lucas, pp.49-71

ISBN 1-59454-828-5

Chapter 3

INTERINDIVIDUAL VARIATIONS IN RESPONSE TO PAIN AND ANALGESICS

Eufemia Jacob*
Baylor College of Medicine, Houston, TX
Natalie A. Rasmussen†
College of Nursing, University of Nebraska Medical Center, Omaha, NE

ABSTRACT

Clinical observations have shown that wide variations in response to analgesics exist. Some individuals exhibit unrelieved pain despite high doses and others exhibit side effects even with low doses. The effectiveness and side effects of analgesics may be related to the dose, route, and time of administration, as well as genetic factors that may predispose individual variations in response to pain and analgesics. Several studies have examined the rhythms of various types of pain and neuropeptides associated with pain. This chapter will review evidence from the literature, including human and animal studies, that suggests that variations in response to pain and analgesics may be explained by rhythmic, pharmacokinetic, and genetic factors that affect the metabolism of and response to analgesics. There will be two major sections to the chapter: 1) Rhythmic variations in mechanisms involved in pain and analgesia and 2) Pharmacokinetic variations in metabolism and disposition of analgesics. Both of these sections will discuss genetic factors that may influence individual responses to pain and analgesics. The roles of these variations need to be thoroughly investigated. Theoretically, potential development of analgesics and individualized dosage regimens for patients with pain may be based on these variations.

---

* Research Fellow in Pediatric Oncology, Baylor College of Medicine, Houston, TX; Texas Children's Hospital, Clinical Research Center, 6621 Fannin St, MC1-3320; Houston, TX 77030; Phone (832) 824-4863; Fax (832) 825-6479; e-mail: exjacob@texaschildrenshospital.org

† Assistant Professor, College of Nursing, University of Nebraska Medical Center, 985330 Nebraska Medical Center, Omaha, NE 68198-5330; Office: CON, Room 5034; Phone (402) 559-9758; Fax (402) 559-4303; e-mail: nrasmuss@unmc.edu

INTRODUCTION

The body of evidence demonstrating differences in analgesic response to various analgesics is progressively increasing. The sequencing of the human genome [1, 2] stimulated research interests on the search for pharmacogenetic predictors of individual responses to analgesics. Animal models are being developed to examine the allelic variants that underlie the genetic sources of variability in pain experiences and analgesic responses. Genetic polymorphisms were regarded as genetic causes for changes in the rhythmicity of biological processes and the pharmacokinetics of analgesics. This review will summarize the evidence that genetic variations may contribute to the variations in rhythmicity that affect pain and analgesics and genetic variations that may affect differences in analgesic efficacy and/or potency. The first section will provide general information related to the rhythmic and genetic variations in mechanisms involved in pain and analgesia. The second section will examine genetic variations in pharmacokinetics that affect response to analgesics.

RHYTHMIC AND GENETIC VARIATIONS IN MECHANISMS INVOLVED IN PAIN AND ANALGESIA

Chronobiology

Living organisms developed a biological clock in order to allow for adaptation to one's environment. One important aspect of the environment that must be adapted to on a daily basis is the light and dark cycle that occurs as the earth rotates. Chronobiology is the study of rhythms in living organisms [3, 4] that have periods of less than five minutes to a lifetime. Three classic theories of biologic circadian rhythms have been proposed [5]. One model states that there is only one pacemaker that drives circadian rhythms. Due to the evidence of adrenal glands and liver cells functioning as oscillators, this model is not widely accepted.

A second model states that organisms have a circadian timing system (CTS) made up of structures in the nervous system that maintain timing of physiological processes and behavior [6]. The CTS consists of photoreceptor cells and projections of the retina or entrainment pathways, circadian pacemakers, and pathways that connect the pacemakers with the effector systems [5]. A *zeitgeber*, or time giver, such as light, dictates the timing of a function. This *zeitgeber* is detected by the retina and transmitted via the retinohypothalamic tract (RHT) to the suprachiasmatic nucleus (SCN). The SCN is the primary pacemaker of this system. It is located in the preoptic-anterior hypothalamus. Impulses may be transmitted to the intergeniculate leaflet (IGL) from the RHT. The IGL can transmit via the geniculohypothalamic tract to the SCN, neuropeptides, such as neuropeptide Y and gamma aminobutyric acid (GABA). The SCN later transmits the stimuli to individual circadian oscillators. These oscillators then transmit the stimuli to the various circadian systems and a response rhythm is produced.

Melatonin is a substance secreted by the pineal gland. It is known to mediate photoperiodic effects [7], act as a circadian pacemaker [8, 9], and express an overt cycle in mammals. Therefore, this model is based on the idea that there is a single pacemaker with multiple oscillators. It is the most widely accepted of the three models. The third model states that there are multiple pacemakers or oscillators that are stimulated by different *zeitgebers* [5].

Clock genes code for proteins that influence rhythms, such as circadian rhythms. There are two classes of genes whose rhythmic expression results in circadian rhythms. These include the central clock genes, which drive downstream rhythms, and the clock-regulated genes, which code for aspects of the circadian output system [6, 10-13]. In mammals, such as humans, the circadian locomotor output cycles kaput (CLOCK) and aryl hydrocarbon receptor nuclear translocator-like (BMAL1 or ARNTL) genes provide positive transcriptional drive in a feedback loop by encoding for CLOCK and BMAL1 proteins. In the light, these proteins turn on genes, such as period homolog 1 (PER1), period homolog 2 (PER2), period homolog 3 (PER3), cryptochrome 1 (CRY1) and cryptochrome 2 (CRY2). These genes provide a negative feedback. The PER and CRY mRNA enters the cytoplasm. The PER and CRY proteins form complexes, enter the nucleus, and function in turning off the PER and CRY genes. The CRY proteins act on CLOCK and/or BMAL1 to inhibit transcription. The PER protein functions also by inhibiting the gene that inhibits BMAL1. This, in turn, increases the level of BMAL1 protein. This process cycles throughout the day.

The clock genes may entrain other genes. For example, in a study using microarray, a number of genes were found to have a variation in expression that was based on time of day [14]. A mutation in these genes may lead to pathological conditions because the rhythm for a body process may be disrupted. Little is known about the effect of a clock gene on the various genes associated with pain and analgesia. Liu and colleagues [15] reported that dependence on morphine in mice was related to the expression of mPer1. Ammon and colleagues [16] studied the effect of chronic morphine on various genes. They found that rPer2 expression was changed.

There are a number of genes of interest to those who study pain and analgesia. Little, however, is known about the circadian influence on these genes. For example, ATP binding cassette (abc) genes are important in drug transportation and code for P-glycoprotein [17]. There are the enzyme genes such as COMT or catechol-O-methyltransferase [18]. Environmental light changes have been noted to have an influence on COMT expression [19]. The gene CYP, with variants 1A,2C, 2D, 2E, and 3A, code for cytochrome P450 enzymes [20, 21]. Some of the CYP genes were found to be unresponsive to circadian influence [22]. The UDP glycosyltransferase 1 family and 2 family (UGT1 and UGT2) genes code for enzymes as well [23]. Karwa and colleagues [24] indicated that there was a circadian influence on the enzymes related to UGT. Genes associated with receptors include, adrenergic receptor, alpha 2a (Adra2a) [25], Htr1b or 5-hydroxytryptamine (serotonin) receptor 1B [26], Mc1r or melanocortin 1 receptor [27], OPRD1 or opioid receptor, delta 1 [28] OPRK or opioid receptor, kappa 1 [29], and Oprm or opioid receptor, mu 1 [30-34]. Knowing the effect that clock genes have on the pain- and analgesia-related genes may assist in the timing and dosing of analgesics so that they are more effective and have fewer side effects.

It is known that prostaglandins [35, 36], natural killer (NK) cells [37], proopiomelanocortin (POMC) and POMC-derived peptides [38-45], met-enkephalin [46], and membrane potentials in neurons [47] have circadian rhythms. It also is known that a stressor, such as surgery, can change or completely abolish the circadian rhythm of biochemicals such as beta-endorphin [48]. Various conditions, such as iron deficiency, cold sensitivity in teeth, biliary pain, headaches, rheumatoid arthritis, and chest pain also can cause a change in the endogenous rhythms [49-57].

A noxious stimulus, such as a hot-plate, was found to cause an alteration in the rhythm of beta-endorphin in mice [43]. Some medications, such as anesthetics and analgesics, have been shown to interfere with the release of biochemicals, such as beta-endorphin. These medications include buprenorphine [58], indomethacin [59], fentanyl [60], and morphine [61]. Having knowledge about an individual's endogenous rhythms and how they are changed by a painful stimulus, pathology, or medication will assist in individualizing the treatment of pain.

Chronopharmacology

In the early 1950s, the influence of rhythms on drug disposition and response was investigated. This became known as chronopharmacology [3, 4, 62, 63]. It is based on the timing of the administration of medication in order to increase its effectiveness or decrease its side effects. It also assists in understanding the periodic changes in desired effects and tolerance [64]. It encompasses the concepts of chronokinetics, chronesthesy, chronergy, and chronotherapy.

Drugs exert a different effect at different times of day because of the time variations in drug absorption, plasma protein binding, drug distribution and metabolism, hepatic blood flow, and in metabolizing enzyme activities [65]. Some of these processes have been found to vary during a 24-hour day [66-74]. Some analgesics have been found to be more effective at certain times of day. For example, indomethacin was noted to be most effective in the early rest period in mice [75]. This was thought to be similar to what is seen in humans with nocturnal pain. Another study reported that morphine effectiveness varied in a 24-hour day [61].

The appearance of the effect of the drug depends on the stage of a programmed function occurring when a drug reaches the target cell [64]. Also, it depends on the rhythm of receptor binding [76]. Food intake may influence the rhythm of drug absorption and gene expression [4, 77]. The gender, age, and health of an individual may also affect drug absorption [4, 64, 78]. Posture and exercise influence the effect of drugs in a day as they are components of rest-sleep and activity-wake states [4]. Also, the genetic make up of the individual should be considered as there are differences in, for example, the effectiveness of some drugs between individuals [79-87]. All of these factors must be considered when medications, such as analgesics, are administered.

The challenge is to incorporate what is known about chronopharmacology into the care of clients. Chronotherapy is rarely considered in the treatment of diseases or symptoms. Most medications are administered at a time convenient for the health care professional and/or client. Smolensky [88] noted that physicians may need more education regarding treatments around the clock. They may not have knowledge about how to prescribe a medication so that it is effective at all times of the day and has fewer side effects. On the other hand, the issue may not be the lack of knowledge. It may, perhaps, be due to an unwillingness to change current practice.

It would seem that administering different dosages of a medication at different times of day would be more complex. The outcome of treatment, however, may be improved. If so, it would be worth the time and effort to implement treatment based on time of day. For example, Gourlay and colleagues [68] examined the potential mismatch between fluctuations in pain intensity and morphine blood concentrations as a consequence of chronopharmacokinetic variability for morphine administered orally. They found differences in the maximum concentration of morphine that were dependent on time of morphine administration during the day. They attributed their findings to the possible changes in the rate of gastric emptying, which was demonstrated to have circadian variability [89]. It is possible that chronopharmacokinetic variability may affect the absorption, metabolism, volume of distribution, and protein binding of morphine, so that the analgesic effects may depend on the timing of morphine administration. Because morphine is extensively metabolized by the liver, the circadian changes in the hepatic blood flow [90] and the diurnal variability in enzyme activity [65] may affect the achievement of plasma concentrations that depend on the time of day.

Pharmacogenetics

A goal for pain management in the future would be to have an understanding of genetics and pain and analgesic mechanisms that would allow for the development of an algorithm for the individualized administration of analgesics to optimize the beneficial effects of analgesics and decrease the adverse effects throughout a 24-hour day. Individualized medicine is being considered in the treatment of diseases such as colorectal cancer [91], hypertension [92], and atherosclerosis [93]. Gene therapy also is being considered as a possible treatment for pain [94-96]. However, over all, the current management of diseases and symptoms is not individualized. The use of microarray analysis can be used clinically to provide information about an individual's gene expression patterns [97]. Samples for microarray should be collected at least every 4 hours in order to determine the circadian influence on genes. Outcomes of the treatment could be determined by monitoring treatment-induced changes in the gene expression patterns. This will assist in determining the most effective and least harmful treatment of pain around the clock.

Genetic Variations in Pharmacokinetics that Affect Response to Analgesics

Response to analgesics in terms of pain relief and adverse effects are currently being attributed to genetic variability. Analgesics may have no effect because medications may be rapidly cleared from the body as a result of duplication or amplification of genes for enzymes that metabolize them. Analgesics also may produce toxic side effects as a result of sub-or non-functional genes for enzymes, which are unable to metabolize certain drugs. Both of these situations are linked to certain genetic polymorphisms, which may lead to the overexpression and underexpression of genes that cause the lack of activity, a decreased activity, or an increased activity in the enzymes that metabolize analgesics.

Genes with variations in expression include the cytochrome P450 (CYPs), glutathione sulfotransferases (GSTs)-transferases, and Uridine diphosphate-glucuronyl transferases (UGT's) that are relevant to the metabolism and toxicology of analgesics. However, cellular signaling pathways leading to toxicity are not thoroughly characterized and genes involved in drug response pathways have not been identified [98]. Advances in microarray technology may be able to identify appropriate gene sets that would elucidate these mechanisms and pathways [99]. Expression patterns generated by "no observed adverse effect level" or "lowest observed adverse effect level" need to be compared to determine whether genes and pathways are activated at the non-toxic, toxic and lethal doses [98]. Single nucleotide polymorphisms (SNP) in the protein coding sequences of genes are estimated to be around 200-300,000. Characterizing them may explain individual variations in drug absorption, drug metabolism, drug interactions with receptors, and how they relate to response.

Cytochrome P40

The cytochrome P450 (CYP) family of genes has multiple variants that are responsible for a high proportion of observed variations in drug response. The liver is a primary site for drug and hormone metabolism. It coordinates not only energy metabolism but also a variety of exocrine and endocrine functions. The CYP genes are regulated within the liver in response to diet, xenobiotics, and hormonal balance. There are three drug metabolizing enzymes that process analgesics in the liver. These drug metabolizing enzymes 1) modify substrates directly via oxidation, hydroxylation, and dealkylation (Phase I enzymes); 2) conjugate drugs to sulfate, glutathion, or carbohydrates to facilitate clearance (Phase II enzymes), and 3) directionally transport these conjugates from liver into the bile or urine (Phase III enzymes). The CYP family (CYP2D, CYP2C, CYP4A) collectively metabolize approximately 90% of drugs [99]. Genetic variations in these enzymes can influence the pharmacokinetics and pharmacology of analgesics, which may lead to profound toxicity or reduced efficacy of analgesics metabolized by these polymorphic enzymes. Characterization of these genetic variations in these enzymes will eventually explain why analgesics work better in some individuals than they do in others.

CYP2D6

The cytochrome P4502D6 (CYP2D6) plays an important role in the metabolism of drugs, including morphine derivatives and antidepressant agents. The CYP2D6 is highly polymorphic with over 70 known variants, leading to wide variations in CYP2D6 enzyme activity, from ultrarapid metabolizer to poor metabolizer phenotypes. Approximately 9.8% of Caucasians were characterized as poor metabolizers, while a significant proportion (30%) of black American subjects were characterized as poor metabolizers [100]. Because data for dosing guidelines were derived from studies conducted solely in Caucasian subjects, clinicians need to pay attention to ethnic differences in drug response. Dosing adjustments of analgesic regimens may be required in designing therapeutic approaches in black Americans and other non-Caucasians. Compared with Caucasians, black Americans showed higher median dextromethorphan/dextrorphan ratio, which is consistent with overall slower CYP2D6 activity toward dextromethorphan [100, 101].

Pharmacogenetic differences have been observed within each ethnic group that determines susceptibility to the extremes of response (e.g. lack of efficacy at one end of the spectrum and excessive toxicity at the other end).

The allelic variants that determine the poor metabolizer status extreme of the black Americans may be different from those that identify a poor metabolizer among Caucasians

[100]. The most commonly observed null alleles among Caucasians were 2D6*3, 2D6*4, 2D6*5, and 2D6*6, which accounts for only 2 of the 14 poor metabolizers among black Americans. The intermediate metabolizers among the black Americans showed that the 2D6*17 and 2D6*29 alleles were overrepresented in this group compared with the extensive metabolizers. These two alleles were observed very rarely in Caucasian subjects. Slower phenotypes were observed among black Americans with the 2D6*1/*1, 2D6*1/*2, or 2D6*2/*2, when compared with the Caucasian subjects who had the same genotypes.

The difference in phenotypes despite same genotypes have been attributed to polymorphic variations in the CYP2D6 regulatory regions, but these require further validation [100]. The assignment of CYP2D6 status in a given black American individual was based on Caucasian derived criteria. Caucasian subjects who were characterized as poor metabolizers (dextromethorphan/ dextrorphan metabolic ratio >0.3) were generally considered to be at a higher risk for development of concentration-dependent adverse drug reactions compared with extensive metabolizers. However, the values for black Americans (for example, ratio > 0.4) that define the extensive metabolizers and poor metabolizers may be different than the values that were used to characterize them in Caucasian subjects [100].

In the Mexican American population, the frequency distribution of poor metabolizers is approximately 3.2%, which lies between the frequencies noted for Asian and Caucasian populations [102]. The clinical consequences of CYP2D6 activities may affect responsiveness to analgesics. For example, in a study that examined differences in response to postoperative tramadol analgesia after an abdominal surgery [103], poor metabolizers associated with CYP2D6 mutations displayed a higher rate of non-response, consumed 30% more tramadol, and required additional rescue medications than extensive metabolizers. The risk for concentration-dependent toxicities may be different for different populations, which may affect the effectiveness of analgesics and may explain variations in their responses to the amount and dosing intervals of analgesic regimens.

CYP2C19

The cytochrome P450 2C's (CYP2C) are an important subfamily of P450 enzymes that metabolize approximately 20% of clinically used drugs, including nonsteroidal anti-inflammatory drugs, the anxiolytic agent diazepam, and other drugs used for management of neuropathic pain, such as antidepressants and anticonvulsants [104]. Diazepam is demethylated by CYP2C19. Variations in the plasma half-life of diazepam were demonstrated to be dramatically different depending on genotypes. The plasma half-life of individuals genotyped as homozygous for the defective CYP2C19*2 allele was longer (84 hours) than either individuals who were homozygous for the wild-type CYP2C19*1 allele (20 hours), or individuals heterozygous for one defective CYP2C19 allele (64 hours) [105, 106]. Asian populations have been reported to have slower metabolism of diazepam than Caucasians, which may be attributed to the higher frequency of the mutant CYP2C19*2 and CYP2C19*3 alleles among Asians [107]. Clinicians need to pay attention to the dosing of poor metabolizers because toxic doses of diazepam may occur as the result of slower metabolism.

CYP2C9

CYP2C9 metabolizes the anticonvulsant phenytoin. Individuals homozygous for CYP2C9*3 allele have decreased clearance of phenytoin. Clinical problems with toxicity and dosage adjustment have been found in CYP2C9 poor metabolizers [108, 109]. CYP2C9 accounts for 80-90% of the metabolism of phenytoin. Therefore, polymorphisms in CYP2C9 have a larger effect on the clinical toxicity of phenytoin. The recombinant CYP2C9*3 also has a higher K*m* (the concentration of drug at half-maximum rate of metabolism) for the nonsteroidal anti-inflammatory drug (NSAID) diclofenac 4'hydroxylation and a lower V*max* (maximum rate of metabolism) for the NSAIDs piroxicam 5'-hydroxylation, tenoxicam 5'-hydroxylation, mefenamic acid 3'-hydroxylation, which resulted in lower intrinsic clearance values for the CYP2C9 substrates [110]. In some cases, the effect may alter the affinity of the enzyme for the substrates and in other cases, the mutations affect the V*max*. Individuals who are homozygous for CYP2C9*3 may have slower metabolism of these drugs, but the clinical consequences have not been examined. The CYP2C9 poor metabolizer has a frequency of approximately 6% in Caucasians and the frequency of the homozygous CYP2C9*3 poor metabolizer is approximately 0.3% [111].

CYP2C9 and Ibuprofen

Ibuprofen, a nonselective inhibitor of cyclooxygenases 1 and 2 (COX-1 and COX-2) contains the racemic mixture of R9-) and S-(+)-ibuprofen that are eliminated after oxidative biotransformation and glucuronidation in the liver [112]. The population clearance of individuals with the CYP2C9*3/*3 genotype was 2.37 L/h, which was about 50% lower than that of individuals with the CyP2C9*1/*1 genotype (3.77 L/h) [113]. The elimination half-lives of racemic ibuprofen were significantly different between the CYP2C9*1/*1 (2.04 hours) and CYP2C9*3/*3 genotypes (3.09 hours). The magnitude of the area under the plasma concentration-time curve (AUC) and the measured maximal plasma concentrations (C*max*) of racemic ibuprofen and of S-ibuprofen were higher in individuals with the CYP2C9 slow genotypes [113]. The AUC values of racemic ibuprofen and S-ibuprofen were almost twice as high in individuals with CYP2C9*3/*3 genotype when compared with individuals with CYP2C9*1/*1 genotype. The median plasma concentrations of the 2-hydroxyibuprofen-metabolites generated by CYP2C9 was lower in carriers of the *3/*3 genotype than individuals of other genotypes. The prolonged half-life of ibuprofen in individuals with the *3/*3 resulted in a prolonged inhibition of thromboxane B_2 formation. The duration of the 50% inhibition of cyclooxygenases 1 was longer in individuals of the slow metabolic genotypes. The duration of 50% inhibition was significantly longer in individuals with CYP2C9 genotypes *2/*3 (14 hours) and genotypes *3/*3 (20 hours), when compared with individuals with the wildtype genotype [113].

A number of other NSAIDs were identified as substrates of cytochrome P450 2C9 including indomethacin [114], flurbiprofen [115, 116], naproxen [117], piroxicam [118], lornoxicam [119], mefenamic acid, and meloxicam [120]. However, clinical studies have not validated their effects on metabolism, analgesia and toxicity. In a study that examined the influences of the known amino acid variants, CYP2C9*2 (Arg144Cys) and CYP2C9*3 (Ile359Leu), on diclofenac pharmacokinetics after a 50 mg oral dose of diclofenac, there was no evidence of impaired metabolism in healthy individuals who were heterozygous or homozygous when compared with the wildtype [121].

CYP2C9 and Diclofenac

Oral clearance of diclofenac varied about four-fold, with a mean value of 27.2 liter/hour. There was a more than 10-fold variability in the maximal diclofenac plasma concentrations (C*max*) with a mean of 1.7 mg/liter. Plasma concentrations of the metabolite 4'-

hydroxydiclofenac were not lower in individuals with the CYP2C9 low activity alleles *2 and *3 compared with the individuals of CYP2C9 *1/ *1 genotype. The plasma concentration-time courses from individuals with the homozygous CYP2C9 genotypes *1 /*1, *2/ *2, and *3 /*3 did not show significant diclofenac concentrations [121].

A large decline in serum thromboxane B_2 (TxB_2) concentrations was seen about 1-2 hours after dosing [121]. Marked diclofenac-mediated inhibition of Cox-1 and Cox-2 activity was detected in all individuals independent of CYP2C9 genotype. A steep decline in plasma prostaglandin E_2 (PGE_2) was seen about 1 hour after diclofenac intake. PGE_2 concentrations at baseline (before medication) varied more than 15-fold. After administration of diclofenac, inhibition was detected throughout the decline in diclofenac concentrations. Concentrations of PGE_2 did not depend on CYP2C9 genotypes.

Other studies were unable to detect a significant difference in the diclofenac total clearance among healthy heterozygous individuals with the CYP2C9 *1/*3 genotype compared with the homozygous wildtypes [122-125]. However, these studies were conducted with small sample sizes and with healthy individuals. Larger samples may have the power to detect significance. Also, if studies were conducted in individuals with altered physiological states, significant differences in effects may be found with variations in genotypes. The mean total clearance of diclofenac in individuals with the genotype CYP2C9 *1/*3 (n=4) was about 60%. In heterozygous for CYP2C9 *1/*2 (n=3) the mean total clearance was about 80% of the clearance in individuals with the wild-type genotype CYP2C9 *1/*1. An increase in the metabolic ratio of diclofenac /4'-OH diclofenac in heterozygous carriers of the alleles *3 and *2 compared with individuals with homozygous wild type was detected in one study, but may not have reached statistical significance due to a small sample [122].

Uridine Diphospate-Glucuronyl Transferases (UGT's)

The uridine diphosphate (UDP)-glucuronosyltransferase (UGT) enzymes play a central role in the biotransformation of many medications in the liver, including morphine. UGT gene variants affect the disposition of the substrates of glucuronidation and may potentially increase the variability in pharmacokinetics [126].

Morphine and UGT2B7

Morphine is metabolized to morphine-3-glucoronide (M3G) and morphine-6-glucoronide (M6G). With high doses of morphine, the accumulation of these metabolites may be associated with an increased risk for side effects [127-130] and paradoxical pain [129], in which increasing doses of morphine appear to generate worsening pain behavior and agitation. Morphine-6-glucuronide (M6G) is an active metabolite [131]. M6G is a much more potent analgesic than morphine itself, and has significant analgesic activity [132]. Approximately 90% of a given dose is conjugated to morphine-6-glucuronide (M6G) and morphine-3-glucuronide (M3G) [131]. M6G appears in serum approximately 6 minutes after intravenous administration [133]. Peak plasma levels of M6G are about one-fourth of those of morphine after intravenous dosing.

Morphine is metabolized by the liver microsomes by N-demethylation, N-dealkylation, O-dealkylation, conjugation and hydrolysis. The majority of clearance is by hepatic glucuronidation, such as morphine-3-glucuronide (50%) and M6G (5 to 15%). The ability to metabolize morphine into M3G and M6G varies substantially between individuals. Genetic polymorphisms of morphine glucuronidation has been considered as a possible cause. Uridine diphosphate-glucuronosyltransferase 2B7 (UGT2B7) is the major enzyme responsible for the 3-and 6-glucuronidation of morphine in humans. A polymorphism in the gene expressing the UGT2B7 enzyme has been identified that consists of a C-to-T point mutation. This point mutation resulted in an amino acid change from histidine (H) to tyrosine (Y) at amino acid 268, which is the proposed location of the substrate-binding site [134, 135].

In a study that investigated the variation in the UGT2B7 gene in postoperative patients receiving patient controlled analgesia with morphine, M6G:morphine ratios were stratified by genotype [126]. A significant trend for decreased M6G:morphine ratios was observed in Caucasian patients with T/T (medial value 1.0), C/T (median value 0.81), and C/C (median value 0.59;p=0.031) genotypes. Genotype explained 6.6% of the variation in M6G:morphine ratios (p=0.038). The same trend also was observed for M3G:morphine ratios, but statistical significance was not reached, most likely because of small sample size (p=0.055).

A significant trend for median values of morphine concentrations also was observed for patients with C/C (mean 68 ng/ml), C/T (mean 63 ng/ml), and T/T (18 ng/ml) genotypes. Morphine concentrations were significantly lower in T/T patients than in C/T and C/C patients (p=0.04). For M3G concentrations the median values were 152 ng/l (C/C), 259 ng/ml (C/T), and 203 ng/ml (T/T). For M6G, the median values were 18 ng/ml, 46 ng/ml, and 18 ng/ml, respectively. M6G and M3G concentrations were significantly lower in C/C patients than in C/T (p=0.045) and T/T (p=0.004) patients. A significant overall difference in M6G concentration across genotypes was observed (p=0.0085), but no statistical difference was observed for morphine and M3G levels [126].

The clinical significance in these variations need to be investigated. In a case report that presented two patients with very different clinical responses to morphine (sensitive and low responder), the nucleotide sequence of UGT2B7 and the genotype patterns between the two patients were remarkably different [136]. Cancer patient 1, with hypopharyngeal cancer suffering from severe neck pain due to cervical lymph node metastasis, was administered 10 mg of morphine via a slow release table daily. Two days later, severe drowsiness and confusion developed. The side effects disappeared after withdrawal of the morphine slow release tablet. Patient 2, with a Pancoast tumor suffering from severe pain in the left shoulder and upper chest wall due to metastases in the third rib, was administered up to 2000 mg daily. The pain was not relieved and no side effects were observed. Remarkable differences in the nucleotide sequence were observed between the patients. Patient 1 had reference alleles at several SNP positions and a rare homozygous ATTGAT*2C sequence. Patient 2 had the predominant homozygous GCCAGC*1G sequence.

In a study by Holthe and colleagues [137] that investigated whether polymorphisms in UGT2B7 contributes to the variability in morphine glucuronide to morphine plasma ratios among cancer patients undergoing analgesic therapy with morphine, the M3G and M6G to morphine plasma ratios varied 16 to 42 fold between individuals. However, no correlation was seen between UGT2B7 genotypes and M3G:morphine and M6G: morphine ratios [137].

Serum concentrations of morphine, M6G, and M3G obtained during clinical routine drug monitoring in patients with cancer, did not have a direct concentration-effect relationship with pain intensity, nausea, tiredness, cognitive function or constipation [138-140]. Patients with morphine-resistant pain had similar M3G concentrations as patients with well-controlled pain [141]. There is conflicting data regarding the relationship between the serum concentration of

M3G and M6G in patients with confusion. Ashby and colleagues [128] reported a higher concentration of M3G and M6G in patients with confusion than for patients without this adverse effect. However, Tiseo and colleagues [130] found no significant differences in morphine and M6G concentrations between patients with confusion and patients who did not have confusion. In these studies, only a small numbers of patients were studied. In addition, wide variability of events and other patient-related factors, such as pain mechanisms, antitumor treatments, metabolic status, hydration, and severity and localization of the cancer [139] may explain the inconsistency in findings.

Morphine and Mu Opioid Receptor Gene

The human mu-opioid receptor is the major site for the analgesic action for most of the opioid analgesics, such as morphine. Morphine is not analgesic without functioning mu-opioid receptors. The individual differences in response to morphine were believed to be at least partly caused by genetic variations in the mu-opioid receptors. Studies of mice showed that if the mice did not have mu opioid receptors, their threshold for pain was much lower and they did not respond to mu opioid analgesics like morphine [142]. The human gene encoding the mu opioid receptor has been cloned and physically mapped to the chromosomal region 6q24-125 [143]. Mutation screening of the coding and 5' regulatory regions has revealed several DNA sequence variants [144-146]. The most prevalent single-nucleotide polymorphism is a nucleotide exchange at position 118 (A118G). An amino acid substitution of aspargine to aspartic acid (Asn40Asp) in the extracellular N-terminal domain at a high conserved N-glycosylation site was predicted [144, 147], which was shown to have a three times higher affinity to beta endorphin. Genotypes in the mu opioid receptor gene may explain individual differences in response to morphine.

Large interindividual variations in the serum concentrations of morphine, morphine-6-glucruronide (M6G), and morphie-3-glucuronide (M3G) were observed in patients receiving chronic morphine therapy [128, 148-151]. While M6G contributes to the analgesic effects of morphine [149, 152], the clinical effects from M3G as it relates to the potential for eliciting neurotoxic effects have been disputed [153, 154]. The ratios M3G:morphine and M6G:morphine were lower in patients receiving morphine by parenteral routes compared with the oral route. These differences were related to variations in both first-pass metabolism and elimination. The first-pass effect is disregarded during parenteral administration of morphine, thereby allowing a larger fraction of the variability to be determined by variations in renal elimination. The differences in the M3G:morphine and M6G:morphine ratios were higher with the accumulation of M6G and M3G for those patients with renal failure [150, 155, 156]. However, in patients with normal renal function, individual patient characteristics were found to predict only minor parts of the variability of morphine, M3G and M6G serum concentrations observed during routine clinical drug monitoring [138, 150, 157].

In 207 patients using morphine for malignant disease, patients who reported adequate pain control were predominantly homozygous wild-type (n=78) and some were heterozygous for the 118 A>G polymorphism, a few (n=4) were homozygous for the variant 118 G allele. Pain intensity was significantly different between groups, with the patients heterozygous for the 118A > G polymorphism having more pain [158]. The patients homozygous for the 118 G allele received significantly higher daily morphine doses compared to the wild-type patients. The serum concentrations of morphine, M6G and M3G showed significantly higher clinical results in patients homozygous for the 118 G allele. Morphine may have decreased efficacy in patients with 118 G allele, which may be attributed to decreased efficacy of M6G in individuals heterozygous or homozygous for the 118 A>G OPRM1 gene. M6G is transported slowly through the blood brain barrier and has little effect after short term administrations [132, 159]. During chronic morphine administration, however, genetic variability in M6G efficacy influenced morphine efficacy [158]. Such variability may contribute to the variable analgesic effect and tolerance for opioids in individuals [160, 161].

Mu Opioid Receptor Gene and Splice Variants

The concept of multiple mu opioid receptors was proposed over 20 years ago [162]. Most of the opioids used clinically are mu-selective and clinicians have observed differences among these drugs. Some patients respond far better to one mu opioid than another with respect to analgesia and side effects. One opioid may be a superior analgesic in one patient, while a different mu opioid may be better in another patient. Side effects also vary, with some individuals unable to tolerate morphine due to nausea and vomiting, but may be able to tolerate another mu opioid such as methadone without a problem.

Individuals who are highly tolerant to one opioid may be rotated to a different opioid [163]. Relative potencies of different mu opioids in highly tolerant individuals are not the same as in individuals who are opioid naïve. When rotated to another opioid, the individual may show far less tolerance and may receive analgesia at a relative lower dose. The dose of the second mu opioid is commonly calculated at 50-75% lower from the equivalency tables determined from naïve patients. Genetic influences on variations in response to analgesics have been extensively studied and are well established in mice, with sensitivity and relative potency variations within and between strains [164-166].

A large number of mu opioid receptor (MOR-1) variants have been identified in mice [32-34, 167]. All these variants contain exons 1, 2, and 3, which comprise all seven transmembrane domains that form the mu opioid receptor binding pockets. All the variants retain high affinity and selectivity for mu opioids in receptor binding assays. They differ structurally at the region important in transduction of the signal following receptor activation in the C-terminus [168]. The GTPγS maximal stimulation (a measure of efficacy) and the rank order of the efficacy of the mu opioid analgesics varied among the variants. The distribution of the MOR-1 variants within the brain and spinal cord vary, and even if they exist in the same brain region, cell-specific processing has been noted. Cells express either MOR-1 or MOR-C in the dorsal horn of the spinal cord, but not both. MOR-1 may be present both pre- and post-synaptically, but MOR-C is present only presynaptically [169-171].

The complexity of alternative splicing and the differences in location, both within a cell and regionally, may contribute to the variations in individual responses to mu opioid analgesics. Morphine analgesia is downregulated by antisense against exons 6, 7, 8, 9 and 10, as well as exon 4. All antisense targeting each exon can decrease mu analgesia, and morphine analgesia may be mediated by more than one variant. Activation of the different variants would vary significantly based upon the range of efficacies and the wide range of potencies. The actions of mu opioids reflect the activation of all the combined mu opioid receptor variants and the relative contribution to the pharmacologic effect of each splice variant may vary, depending on the potency and efficacy of the analgesics at that particular site [162].

Mu Opioid Receptor Gene Splice Variants and M6G

Mu opioid receptor heterogeneity was implied by the morphine metabolite morphine-6β-glucuronide (M6G), which has long been known to have analgesic activity. M6G was far more potent than morphine when given centrally and accumulated to levels greater than those of morphine in serum of patients [130]. Much of the analgesic response seen clinically may have resulted from the accumulation of M6G, particularly for those patients on chronic morphine treatment. The existence of discrete M6G receptor mechanisms of analgesia have been noted in studies with mice that respond poorly to morphine, but respond normally to M6G [172-175].

The sensitivity profile of morphine differed from M6G. Probes against MOR-1 exons 1 and 4 blocked morphine, but not M6G. While other probes against MOR-1 exons 2 and 3 blocked M6G, but not morphine [176, 177]. MOR variants lacking exons 2 and 3 and other variants lacking exons 1 and 4 have been cloned using a MOR-1 knockout model [174]. In this model, the disruption of exon 1 rendered morphine completely inactive at doses up to 20-fold greater than its ED_{50} in wildtype animals, but M6G retained full analgesic activity.

CONCLUSIONS

This review summarized the evidence that genetic variations may contribute to the variations in rhythmicity that affect pain and analgesics and genetic variations that may affect differences in analgesic efficacy and/or potency. The roles of these variations in individual responses to pain and analgesics need to be thoroughly investigated. By considering rhythmic, pharmacokinetic, and genetic variations, it theoretically would be possible to develop individualized dosage regimens for patients with pain.

REFERENCES

[1] Lander, E.S., et al., Initial sequencing and analysis of the human genome. *Nature,* 2001. 409(6822): p. 860-921.

[2] Venter, J.C., et al., The sequence of the human genome. *Science,* 2001. 291(5507): p. 1304-51.

[3] Ritschel, W.A. and H. Forusz, Chronopharmacology: a review of drugs studied. *Methods Find Exp Clin Pharmacol,* 1994. 16(1): p. 57-75.

[4] Wetterberg, L., Light and biological rhythms. *J Intern Med,* 1994. 235(1): p. 5-19.

[5] Moore-Ede, M., F. Sulzman, and C. Fuller, *The Clocks That Time Us.* 1982, Cambridge, MA: Harvard University Press.

[6] Aronson, B.D., et al., Negative feedback defining a circadian clock: autoregulation of the clock gene frequency. *Science,* 1994. 263(5153): p. 1578-84.

[7] Goldman, B.D. and J.M. Darrow, The pineal gland and mammalian photoperiodism. *Neuroendocrinology,* 1983. 37(5): p. 386-96.

[8] Takahashi, J.S. and M. Menaker, Role of the suprachiasmatic nuclei in the circadian system of the house sparrow, Passer domesticus. *J Neurosci,* 1982. 2(6): p. 815-28.

[9] Takahashi, J.S. and M. Zatz, Regulation of circadian rhythmicity. *Science,* 1982. 217(4565): p. 1104-11.

[10] Clayton, J.D., C.P. Kyriacou, and S.M. Reppert, Keeping time with the human genome. *Nature,* 2001. 409(6822): p. 829-31.

[11] Green, C.B. and J.C. Besharse, Tryptophan hydroxylase expression is regulated by a circadian clock in Xenopus laevis retina. *J Neurochem*, 1994. 62(6): p. 2420-8.

[12] Hall, J.C., Tripping along the trail to the molecular mechanisms of biological clocks. *Trends Neurosci,* 1995. 18(5): p. 230-40.

[13] Loros, J.J. and J.C. Dunlap, Neurospora crassa clock-controlled genes are regulated at the level of transcription. *Mol Cell Biol*, 1991. 11(1): p. 558-63.

[14] Kita, Y., et al., Implications of circadian gene expression in kidney, liver and the effects of fasting on pharmacogenomic studies. *Pharmacogenetics*, 2002. 12(1): p. 55-65.

[15] Liu, Y., et al., The role of mPer1 in morphine dependence in mice. Neuroscience, 2005. 130(2): p. 383-8.

[16] Ammon, S., et al., Microarray analysis of genes expressed in the frontal cortex of rats chronically treated with morphine and after naloxone precipitated withdrawal. *Brain Res Mol Brain Res*, 2003. 112(1-2): p. 113-25.

[17] Polli, J.W., et al., The systemic exposure of an N-methyl-D-aspartate receptor antagonist is limited in mice by the P-glycoprotein and breast cancer resistance protein efflux transporters. *Drug Metab Dispos*, 2004. 32(7): p. 722-6.

[18] Zubieta, J.K., et al., COMT val158met genotype affects mu-opioid neurotransmitter responses to a pain stressor. *Science,* 2003. 299(5610): p. 1240-3.

[19] Gallara, R.V., et al., Environmental light conditions alter gene expression of rat catecholamine biosynthetic enzymes and Neuropeptide Y: differential effect in superior cervical ganglia and adrenal gland. *Brain Res Mol Brain Res,* 2004. 124(2): p. 152-8.

[20] Donato, M.T. and J.V. Castell, Strategies and molecular probes to investigate the role of cytochrome P450 in drug metabolism: focus on in vitro studies. *Clin Pharmacokinet*, 2003. 42(2): p. 153-78.

[21] Shimada, T., et al., Interindividual variations in human liver cytochrome P-450 enzymes involved in the oxidation of drugs, carcinogens and toxic chemicals: studies with liver microsomes of 30 Japanese and 30 Caucasians. *J Pharmacol Exp Ther*, 1994. 270(1): p. 414-23.

[22] Ling, G., et al., Regulation of cytochrome P450 gene expression in the olfactory mucosa. *Chem Biol Interact,* 2004. 147(3): p. 247-58.

[23] Burchell, B., et al., The UDP glucuronosyltransferase gene superfamily: suggested nomenclature based on evolutionary divergence. *DNA Cell Biol*, 1991. 10(7): p. 487-94.

[24] Karwa, R., et al., Time-dependent pharmacokinetic interaction between zidovudine and rifampicin following oral administration at 10.00 and 22.00 hours. *Drug Metabol Drug Interact*, 2001. 18(2): p. 123-34.

[25] Bailey, K. and A. Gibbons, Towards understanding neural survival, differentiation and death. *Genome Biol,* 2002. 3(7): p. REPORTS4018.

[26] Hain, H.S., J.K. Belknap, and J.S. Mogil, Pharmacogenetic evidence for the involvement of 5-hydroxytryptamine (Serotonin)-1B receptors in the mediation of morphine antinociceptive sensitivity. *J Pharmacol Exp Ther*, 1999. 291(2): p. 444-9.

[27] Mogil, J.S., et al., Identification of a sex-specific quantitative trait locus mediating nonopioid stress-induced analgesia in female mice. *J Neurosci,* 1997. 17(20): p. 7995-8002.

[28] Mogil, J.S., et al., Genetic sensitivity to hot-plate nociception in DBA/2J and C57BL/6J inbred mouse strains: possible sex-specific mediation by delta2-opioid receptors. *Pain,* 1997. 70(2-3): p. 267-77.

[29] Bergeson, S.E., et al., Quantitative trait loci influencing morphine antinociception in four mapping populations. *Mamm Genome*, 2001. 12(7): p. 546-53.

[30] Bergen, A.W., et al., Mu opioid receptor gene variants: lack of association with alcohol dependence. *Mol Psychiatry*, 1997. 2(6): p. 490-4.

[31] Crowley, J.J., et al., A genetic association study of the mu opioid receptor and severe opioid dependence. *Psychiatr Genet*, 2003. 13(3): p. 169-73.

[32] Pan, X., et al., Identification and characterization of three new alternatively spliced mu opioid receptor isoforms. *Mol Pharmacol*, 1999. 56: p. 396-403.

[33] Pan, X., et al., Isolation and expression of a novel alternatively spliced mu opioid receptor isoform, MOR-1F. *FEBS Lett,* 2000. 466: p. 337-340.

[34] Pan, Y., et al., Generation of the mu opioid receptor (MOR-1) protein by three new splice variants of the Oprm gene. *Proc Natl Acad Sci,* 2001. 98: p. 14084-14089.

[35] Tracey, D.J. and J.S. Walker, Pain due to nerve damage: are inflammatory mediators involved? *Inflamm Res*, 1995. 44(10): p. 407-11.

[36] Traynor, K., et al., A pharmacist's primer on chronotherapeutics. *Am Pharm*, 1992. NS32(3): p. 77-83.

[37] Mozzanica, N., et al., Association between circadian rhythms of endogenous hypothalamic opioid peptides and of natural killer cell activity. *Int J Immunopharmacol,* 1991. 13(2-3): p. 317-21.

[38] Gibson, M.J., et al., Circadian variation of beta-endorphin-like immunoreactivity in neurointermediate pituitary. *Peptides,* 1983. 4(3): p. 305-9.

[39] Iranmanesh, A., et al., Circadian, ultradian, and episodic release of beta-endorphin in men, and its temporal coupling with cortisol. *J Clin Endocrinol Metab,* 1989. 68(6): p. 1019-26.

[40] Jamali, A.K. and G. Tramu, Daily cycle of fos expression within hypothalamic POMC neurons of the male rat. *Brain Res,* 1997. 771(1): p. 45-54.

[41] Millington, W.R., et al., A diurnal rhythm in proopiomelanocortin messenger ribonucleic acid that varies concomitantly with the content and secretion of beta-endorphin in the intermediate lobe of the rat pituitary. *Endocrinology,* 1986. 118(2): p. 829-34.

[42] Morgan, C., et al., Syrian hamster proopiomelanocortin cDNA cloning and early seasonal changes in testicular expression. *Gen Comp Endocrinol*, 2003. 133(3): p. 353-7.

[43] Rasmussen, N., *Morphine effects on circadian nociception and beta-endorphin.* 2000, University of Nebraska Medical Center: Omaha, Nebraska.

[44] Veldhuis, J.D., et al., Twenty-four-hour rhythms in plasma concentrations of adenohypophyseal hormones are generated by distinct amplitude and/or frequency modulation of underlying pituitary secretory bursts. *J Clin Endocrinol Metab,* 1990. 71(6): p. 1616-23.

[45] Vuolteenaho, O. and J. Leppaluoto, 24-hour pattern of immunoreactive beta-endorphin and adrenocorticotropic hormone (ACTH) in rat plasma and tissues. *Acta Physiol Scand Suppl,* 1984. 537: p. 75-9.

[46] Wesche, D.L. and R.C. Frederickson, Diurnal differences in opioid peptide levels correlated with nociceptive sensitivity. *Life Sci,* 1979. 24(20): p. 1861-7.

[47] Michel, S., et al., Circadian rhythm in membrane conductance expressed in isolated neurons. *Science,* 1993. 259(5092): p. 239-41.

[48] McIntosh, T.K., et al., Prolonged disruption of plasma beta-endorphin dynamics following surgery. *J Surg Res,* 1985. 38(3): p. 210-5.

[49] Bellamy, N., et al., Circadian rhythm in pain, stiffness, and manual dexterity in rheumatoid arthritis: relation between discomfort and disability. *Ann Rheum Dis*, 1991. 50(4): p. 243-8.

[50] Harkness, J.A., et al., Circadian variation in disease activity in rheumatoid arthritis. *Br Med J (Clin Res Ed)*, 1982. 284(6315): p. 551-4.

[51] Kowanko, I.C., et al., Domiciliary self-measurement in the rheumatoid arthritis and the demonstration of circadian rhythmicity. *Ann Rheum Dis,* 1982. 41(5): p. 453-5.

[52] Ostfeld, A.M., The natural history and epidemiology of migraine and muscle contraction headache. *Neurology,* 1963. 2: p. 11-5.

[53] Pollmann, L. and P.H. Harris, Rhythmic changes in pain sensitivity in teeth. *Int J Chronobiol,* 1978. 5(3): p. 459-64.

[54] Rigas, B., et al., The circadian rhythm of biliary colic. *J Clin Gastroenterol,* 1990. 12(4): p. 409-14.

[55] Seres, J., et al., Evidence for daily rhythms of the expression of proopiomelanocortin, interleukin-1-beta and interleukin-6 in adenopituitaries of male long-evans rats: effect of adjuvant arthritis. *Neuroimmunomodulation,* 2004. 11(5): p. 316-22.

[56] Thompson, D.R., J.E. Pohl, and T.W. Sutton, Circadian variation in the frequency of onset of chest pain in elderly patients with acute myocardial infarction. *Age Ageing,* 1992. 21(2): p. 99-102.

[57] Yehuda, S. and M.B. Youdim, *Brain iron: a lesson from animal models.* Am J Clin Nutr, 1989. 50(3 Suppl): p. 618-25; discussion 625-9.

[58] Schmauss, C. and T.L. Yaksh, In vivo studies on spinal opiate receptor systems mediating antinociception. II. Pharmacological profiles suggesting a differential association of mu, delta and kappa receptors with visceral chemical and cutaneous thermal stimuli in the rat. *J Pharmacol Exp Ther,* 1984. 228(1): p. 1-12.

[59] Knepel, W., et al., Inhibition by prostaglandin E2 of the release of vasopressin and beta-endorphin from rat pituitary neurointermediate lobe or medial basal hypothalamus in vitro. *J Endocrinol,* 1985. 106(2): p. 189-95.

[60] Barna, I., Z. Acs, and J.I. Koenig, Effects of Hypnorm (fentanyl) on ACTH/beta-endorphin levels in plasma, pituitary and brain of 10-day old rats. *Life Sci,* 1993. 52(17): p. 1417-24.

[61] Rasmussen, N.A. and L.A. Farr, Effects of morphine and time of day on pain and beta-endorphin. *Biol Res Nurs,* 2003. 5(2): p. 105-16.

[62] Carlsson, A. and F. Serrin, *Time of day as a factor influencing the toxicity of Nikethamide. Acta Pharmacologica*, 1950. *6*: p. 181-186.

[63] Reinberg, A. and F. Halberg, Circadian chronopharmacology. *Annu Rev Pharmacol,* 1971. 11: p. 455-92.

[64] Reinberg, A.E., Concepts in chronopharmacology. *Annu Rev Pharmacol Toxicol,* 1992. 32: p. 51-66.

[65] Belanger, P.M., et al., Diurnal variations in the transferases and hydrolases involved in glucuronide and sulfate conjugation of rat liver. *Drug Metab Dispos,* 1985. 13(3): p. 386-9.

[66] Bapuji, A.T., et al., Time dependent influence of diazepam on the pharmacokinetics of ibuprofen in man. *Drug Metabol Drug Interact*, 1999. 15(1): p. 71-81.

[67] Bruckner, J.V., et al., Mechanisms of circadian rhythmicity of carbon tetrachloride hepatotoxicity. *J Pharmacol Exp Ther*, 2002. 300(1): p. 273-81.

[68] Gourlay, G.K., J.L. Plummer, and D.A. Cherry, Chronopharmacokinetic variability in plasma morphine concentrations following oral doses of morphine solution. *Pain,* 1995. 61(3): p. 375-81.

[69] Inoue, N., K. Imai, and T. Aimoto, Circadian variation of hepatic glutathione S-transferase activities in the mouse. *Xenobiotica,* 1999. 29(1): p. 43-51.

[70] Martin, C., et al., Effect of age and photoperiodic conditions on metabolism and oxidative stress related markers at different circadian stages in rat liver and kidney. *Life Sci,* 2003. 73(3): p. 327-35.

[71] Noshiro, M., et al., Rhythmic expression of DEC1 and DEC2 in peripheral tissues: DEC2 is a potent suppressor for hepatic cytochrome P450s opposing DBP. *Genes Cells*, 2004. 9(4): p. 317-29.

[72] Ren, S., et al., *Regulation of oxysterol 7alpha-hydroxylase (CYP7B1) in the rat.* Metabolism, 2003. 52(5): p. 636-42.

[73] Su, T. and X. Ding, Regulation of the cytochrome P450 2A genes. *Toxicol Appl Pharmacol,* 2004. 199(3): p. 285-94.

[74] Viitala, P., et al., cAMP mediated upregulation of CYP2A5 in mouse hepatocytes. *Biochem Biophys Res Commun*, 2001. 280(3): p. 761-7.

[75] Cui, Y., et al., Evaluation of chronopharmacodynamics of indomethacin by the kaolin-induced pain model in mice. *Chronobiol Int*, 2003. 20(3): p. 473-84.

[76] Naber, D., A. Wirz-Justice, and M.S. Kafka, Circadian rhythm in rat brain opiate receptor. *Neurosci Lett,* 1981. 21(1): p. 45-50.

[77] Hara, S., et al., Involvement of nitric oxide in intracerebroventricular beta-endorphin-induced neuronal release of methionine-enkephalin. *Brain Res,* 1995. 675(1-2): p. 190-4.

[78] Reinberg, A.E. and I.E. Ashkenazi, Interindividual differences in chronopharmacologic effects of drugs: a background for individualization of chronotherapy. *Chronobiol Int,* 1993. 10(6): p. 449-60.

[79] Halsas, M., et al., Morning versus evening dosing of ibuprofen using conventional and time-controlled release formulations. *Int J Pharm*, 1999. 189(2): p. 179-85.

[80] Kest, B., et al., Genetic variation in morphine analgesic tolerance: a survey of 11 inbred mouse strains. *Pharmacol Biochem Behav*, 2002. 73(4): p. 821-8.

[81] Lasagna, L. and H.K. Beecher, The optimal dose of morphine. *J Am Med Assoc,* 1954. 156(3): p. 230-4.

[82] Lotsch, J., et al., The polymorphism A118G of the human mu-opioid receptor gene decreases the pupil constrictory effect of morphine-6-glucuronide but not that of morphine. *Pharmacogenetics,* 2002. 12(1): p. 3-9.

[83] Oliverio, A., C. Castellano, and B.E. Eleftheriou, Morphine sensitivity and tolerance: a genetic investigation in the mouse. *Psychopharmacologia,* 1975. 42(3): p. 219-24.

[84] Shuster, L., et al., A genetic analysis of the response to morphine in mice: analgesia and running. Psychopharmacologia, 1975. 42(3): p. 249-54.

[85] Terner, J.M., et al., Pharmacogenetic analysis of sex differences in opioid antinociception in rats. *Pain,* 2003. 106(3): p. 381-91.

[86] Williams, D.G., A. Patel, and R.F. Howard, Pharmacogenetics of codeine metabolism in an urban population of children and its implications for analgesic reliability. *Br J Anaesth*, 2002. 89(6): p. 839-45.

[87] Wilson, S.G., et al., The heritability of antinociception: common pharmacogenetic mediation of five neurochemically distinct analgesics. *J Pharmacol Exp Th*er, 2003. 304(2): p. 547-59.

[88] Smolensky, M.H., Knowledge and attitudes of American physicians and public about medical chronobiology and chronotherapeutics. Findings of two 1996 Gallup surveys. *Chronobiol Int,* 1998. 15(4): p. 377-94.

[89] Goo, R.H., et al., Circadian variation in gastric emptying of meals in humans. *Gastroenterology,* 1987. 93(3): p. 515-8.

[90] Lemmer, B. and G. Nold, Circadian changes in estimated hepatic blood flow in healthy subjects. *Br J Clin Pharmacol*, 1991. 32(5): p. 627-9.

[91] Yu, H.K., et al., Expression of human apolipoprotein(a) kringles in colon cancer cells suppresses angiogenesis-dependent tumor growth and peritoneal dissemination. *J Gene Med,* 2005. 7(1): p. 39-49.

[92] Turner, S.T. and G.L. Schwartz, Gene markers and antihypertensive therapy. *Curr Hypertens Rep,* 2005. 7(1): p. 21-30.

[93] Seo, D., et al., Gene expression phenotypes of atherosclerosis. *Arterioscler Thromb Vasc Biol,* 2004. 24(10): p. 1922-7.

[94] Finegold, A.A., A.J. Mannes, and M.J. Iadarola, A paracrine paradigm for in vivo gene therapy in the central nervous system: treatment of chronic pain. *Hum Gene Ther,* 1999. 10(7): p. 1251-7.

[95] Hao, S., et al., HSV-mediated gene transfer of the glial cell-derived neurotrophic factor provides an antiallodynic effect on neuropathic pain. *Mol Ther,* 2003. 8(3): p. 367-75.

[96] Wu, C.M., et al., Regulated, electroporation-mediated delivery of pro-opiomelanocortin gene suppresses chronic constriction injury-induced neuropathic pain in rats. *Gene Ther,* 2004. 11(11): p. 933-40.

[97] Chittur, S.V., DNA microarrays: tools for the 21st Century. *Comb Chem High Throughput Screen,* 2004. 7(6): p. 531-7.

[98] Rockett, J.C., Chipping away at the mystery of drug responses. *Pharmacogenomics J,* 2001. 1(3): p. 161-3.

[99] Gerhold, D., et al., Monitoring expression of genes involved in drug metabolism and toxicology using DNA microarrays. *Physiol Genomics*, 2001. 5(4): p. 161-70.

[100] Gaedigk, A., et al., Unique CYP2D6 activity distribution and genotype-phenotype discordance in black Americans. *Clinical Pharmacology & Therapeutics,* 2002. 72(1): p. 76-89.

[101] Leathart, J., et al., CYP2D6 phenotype-genotype relationships in African-Americans and Caucasians in lost Angeles. *Pharmacogenetics*, 1998. 8: p. 529-41.

[102] Mendoza, R., et al., CYP2D6 polymorphism in a Mexican American population. *Clin Pharmacol Ther,* 2001. 70(6): p. 552-60.

[103] Stamer, U.M., et al., Impact of CYP2D6 genotype on postoperative tramadol analgesia. *Pain,* 2003. 105(1-2): p. 231-8.

[104] Goldstein, J., Clinical relevance of genetic polymorphisms in the human CYP2C subfamily. *British Journal of Clinical Pharmacology,* 2001. 52(4): p. 349-355.

[105] Qin, X., et al., Effect of the gene dosage of CgammaP2C19 on diazepam metabolism in Chinese subjects. *Clinical Pharmacology & Therapeutics,* 1999. 66: p. 642-646.

[106] Wan, J., et al., The elimination of diazepam in Chinese subjects is dependent on the mephenytoin oxidation phenotype. *British Journal of Clinical Pharmacology,* 1996. 42: p. 471-474.

[107] Bertilsson, L., Geographical interracial differences in polymorphic drug oxidation: current state of knowledge of cytochromes P450 (CYP) 2D6) and 2C19. *Clinical Pharmacokinetics*, 1995. 29: p. 192-209.

[108] Kidd, R., et al., Pharmacokinetics of chlorpheniramine, phenytoin, glipizide, and nefedipine in an individual homozygous for the CYP2C9*3 allele. *Pharmacogenetics,* 1999. 9: p. 71-80.

[109] Ninomiya, H., et al., Genetic polymorphism of CYP2C subfamily and excessive serum phenytoin concentration with central nervous system intoxication. *Ther Drug Monit,* 2000. 22: p. 230-232.

[110] Takanashi, K., et al., CYP2C9 Ile359 and Leu359 variants: enzyme kinetic study with seven substrates. *Pharmacogenetics,* 2000. 10: p. 95-104.

[111] Sullivan-Klose, T., et al., The role of the CYP2C9-Leu359 allelic variant in the tolbutamide polymorphism. *Pharmacogenetics,* 1996. 6: p. 341-349.

[112] Davies, N., Clinical pharmacokinetics of ibuprofen: the first 30 years. *Clin Pharmacokinet,* 1998. 34: p. 101-54.

[113] Kircheiner, J., I. Meineke, and G. Freytag, Enantiospecific effects of cytochrome P450 2C9 amino acid variants on ibuprofen pharmacokinetics and on the inhibition of cyclooxygenases 1 and 2. *Clinical Pharmacology & Therapeutics,* 2002. 72(1): p. 62-75.

[114] Nakajima, M., et al., Cytochrome P450 2C(catalyzes indomethacin O-demethylation in human liver microsomes. *Drug Metab Dispos,* 1998. 26: p. 261-266.

[115] Tracy, T., et al., Role of cytochrome P450 2C(and an allelic variant in the 4'-hydroxylation of (R)- and (S)-flurbiprofen. *Biochem Pharmacol,* 1995. 49: p. 1269-1275.

[116] Tracy, T., et al., Studies of flurbiprofen 4'hydroxylation: additional evidence suggesting the sole involvement of cytochrome P450 2C9. *Biochem Pharmacol,* 1995. 52: p. 1305-1309.

[117] Tracy, T., et al., Involvement of multiple cytochrome P450 isoforms in naproxen O-demethylation. *Eur J Clin Pharmacol,* 1997. 52: p. 293-298.

[118] Hutzler, J., M. Hauer, and T. Tracy, Dapsone activation of CP2C9-mediated metabolism: evidence for activation of multiple substrates and a two-site model. *Drug Metab Dispos*, 2001. 29: p. 1029-1034.

[119] Bonnabry, P., T. Leemann, and P. Dayer, Role of human liver microsomal CYP2C9 in the biotransformation of lornoxicam. *Eur J Clin Pharmacol,* 1996. 49: p. 305-308.

[120] Chesne, C., et al., Metabolism of meloxicam in human liver involves cytochromes P450 2C9 and 3A4. *Xenobiotica,* 1998. 18: p. 1-13.

[121] Kircheiner, J., et al., *Pharmacokinetics of diclofenac and inhibition of cyclooxygenases 1 and 2: no relationship to the CYP2C9 genetic polymoprhism in humans.* 2002.

[122] Dorado, R., et al., CYP2C9 genotype and diclofenac hydroxylation in a Spanish population. *Pharmacol Toxicol,* 2001. 89: p. 106.

[123] Morin, S., et al., Is diclofenac a valuable CYP2C9 probe in humans? *Eur J Clin Pharmacol,* 2001. 56: p. 793-797.

[124] Shimamoto, J., et al., Lack of differences in diclofenac (a substrate for CYP2C9) pharmacokinetics in healthy volunteers with respect to the single CYP2C9*3 allele. *Eur J Clin Pharmacol,* 2000. 56: p. 65-68.

[125] Yasar, U., et al., The role of CYP2C9 genotype in the metabolism of diclofenac in vivo and in vitro. *Pharmacol Toxicol,* 2001. 89: p. 106.

[126] Sawyer, M., et al., A pharmacogenetic study of uridine diphosphate-glucuronosyltransferase 2B7 in patients receiving morphine. *Clinical Pharmacology & Therapeutics,* 2003. 73: p. 566-574.

[127] Anderson, B.J., A.D. McKee, and N.H. Holford, Size, myths and the clinical pharmacokinetics of analgesia in paediatric patients. *Clin Pharmacokinet,* 1997. 33(5): p. 313-27.

[128] Ashby, M., et al., Plasma morphine and glucuronide (M3G and M6G) concentrations in hospice inpatients. *J Pain Symptom Manage,* 1997. 14: p. 157-167.

[129] Bowsher, D., Paradoxical pain: When metabolites of morphine are in the wrong ratio. *British Medical Journal,* 1993. 306: p. 473-474.

[130] Tiseo, P., et al., Morphine-6-glucuronide concentrations and opioid-related side effects: a survey in cancer pains. *Pain,* 1995. 61: p. 47-54.

[131] Glare, P.A. and T.D. Walsh, Clinical pharmacokinetics of morphine. *Therapeutic Drug Monitor,* 1991. 13: p. 1-23.

[132] Lotsch, J. and G. Geisslinger, Morphine-6-glucuronide: an analgesic of the future? *Clin Pharmacokinet,* 2001. 40(7): p. 485-99.

[133] Osborne, P., B. Chieng, and M. Christie, Morhpine-6-glucuronide has a higher efficacy than morphine as a mu-opioid receptor agonist in the rat locus coeruleus. *British Journal of Pharmacology,* 2000. 131: p. 1422-1428.

[134] Lampe, J., et al., Prevalence of polymorphisms in the human UDP-Glucuronosyltransferase 2B family. *Cancer Epidemiology, Biomarkers & Prevention,* 2000. 9(329-333).

[135] Lotsch, J., et al., Does the A118G polymorphism at the mu-opioid receptor gene protect against morphine-6-glucuronide toxicity? *Anesthesiology,* 2002. 97(4): p. 814-9.

[136] Hirota, T., et al., Sequence variability and candidate gene analysis in two cancer patients with complex clinical outcomes during morphine therapy. *Drug Metab Dispos,* 2003. 5: p. 677-680.

[137] Holthe, M., et al., Morphine glucuronide-to-morphine plasma ratios are unaffected by the UGT2B7H268Y and UGT1A1*28 polymorphisms in cancer patients on chronic morphine therapy. *Eur J Clin Pharmacol,* 2002. 58: p. 353-356.

[138] Klepstad, P., et al., Routine drug monitoring of serum concentrations of morphine, morphine-3-glucuronide and morphine-6-glucuronide do not predict clinical observations in cancer patients. *Palliative Medicine* 2003, 2003. 17: p. 679-687.

[139] Mercadante, S., The role of morphine glucuronides in cancer pain. *Palliat Med,* 1999. 13: p. 95-104.

[140] Somogyi, A., et al., Plasma concentrations and renal clearance of morphine, morphine -3-glucuronide and morphine-6-glucuronide in cancer patients receiving morphine. Clin *Pharmacokinet,* 1993. 24: p. 413-420.

[141] Goucke, C., P. Hackett, and K. Ilett, Concentrations of morphine, morphine-6-glucoronide and morphine-3-glucuronide in serum and cerebrospinal fluid following morphine administration to patients with morphine-resistant pain. *Pain,* 1994. 56: p. 145-149.

[142] Matthes, et al., Loss of morphine-induced analgesia, reward effect and withdrawal symptoms in mice lacking the mu-opioid-receptor gene. *Nature*, 1996. 383(819-823).

[143] Wang, J., et al., Mu opiate receptor: cDNA cloning and expression. *Proc Natl Acad Sci USA,* 1993. 90: p. 10230-10234.

[144] Bergen, A., et al., Mu opioid receptor gene variants: lack of association with alcohol dependence. *Mol Psychiatry,* 1997. 2: p. 490-494.

[145] Hoehe, M., et al., Sequence variability and candidate gene analysis in complex disease: association of mu opioid receptor gene variation with substance dependence. *Hum Mol Genet,* 2000. 9: p. 2895-2908.

[146] Wendel, B. and M. Hoehe, The human mu opioid receptor gene: 5' regulatory and intronic sequences. *J Mol Med,* 1998. 76: p. 515-532.

[147] Bond, C., et al., Single-nucleotide polymorphism in the human mu opioid receptor gene alters B-endorphin binding and activity. *Neurobiology,* 1998. 95: p. 9608-9613.

[148] Faura, C., et al., Systematic review of factors affecting the ratios of morphine and its major metabolites. *Pain,* 1998. 74: p. 43-53.

[149] Klepstad, P., S. Kaasa, and P. Borchgrevink, Start of oral morphine to cancer patients: effective serum morphine concentrations and contribution from morphine-6-glucuronide to the analgesia produced by morphine. *Eur J Clin Pharmacol*, 2000. 55: p. 713-719.

[150] Klepstad, P., et al., Influences on serum concentration of morphine, M6G and M3G during routine clinical drug monitoring: A prospective survey in 300 adult cancer patients. *Acta Anaesthesiol Scand,* 2003. 47: p. 725-731.

[151] McQuay, H., et al., Oral morphine in cancer pain: influences on morphine and metabolite concentration. *Clin Pharmacol Ther*, 1990. 48: p. 236-244.

[152] Portenoy, R., et al., The metabolite morphine-6-glucuronide contributes to the analgesia produced by morphine infusion in patients with pain and normal renal function. *Clin Pharmacol Ther,* 1992. 51: p. 422-431.

[153] Sjogren, P., J. Dragsted, and C. Christensen, Myoclonic spasm during treatment with high doses of intravenous morphine in renal failure. *Acta Anaesthesiol Scand,* 1993. 37: p. 780-782.

[154] Sjogren, P., et al., Is development of hyperalgesia, allodynia and myoclonus related to morphine metabolism during long-term administration? Six case stories. *Acta Anaesthesiol Scand,* 1998. 42: p. 1070-1075.

[155] Peterson, G., C. Randall, and J. Paterson, Plasma levels of morphine and morphine glucuronides in the treatment of cancer pain: relationship to renal function and route of administration. *Eur J Clin Pharmacol*, 1990. 38: p. 121-124.

[156] Portenoy, R., et al., Plasma morphine and morphine-6-glucuronide during chronic morphine therapy for cancer pain: plasma profiles, steady-state concentrations and the consequences of renal failure. *Pain,* 1991. 47: p. 13-19.

[157] Klepstad, P., et al., Day to day variations during clinical drug monitoring of morphine, morphine-3-glucuronide and morphine-6-glucuronide serum concentrations in cancer patients. A prospective observational study. *BMC Clinical Pharmacology,* 2004. 4(7).

[158] Klepstad, P., et al., The 118 A>G polymorphism in the human mu-opioid receptor gene may increase morphine requirements in patients with pain caused by malignant disease. *Acta Anaesthesiol Scand,* 2004. 48: p. 1232-1239.

[159] Lotsch, J., et al., The transfer half-life of morphine-6-glucuronide from plasma to effect site assessed by pupil size measurement in healthy volunteers. *Anesthesiology,* 2001. 95: p. 1329-1338.

[160] Mercadante, S., et al., Switching from morphine to improve analgesia and tolerability in cancer patients: a prospective study. *J Clin Oncol,* 2001. 19: p. 2898-2904.

[161] Stoutz, N.D., E. Bruera, and M. Suarez-Almazor, Opioid rotation for toxicity reduction in terminal cancer patients. *J Pain Symptom Manage,* 1995. 10: p. 378-384.

[162] Pasternak, G., Multiple opiate receptors: deja vu all over again. *Neuropharmacology,* 2004. 47(Supplement 1): p. 312-323.

[163] Cherny, N., et al., Strategies to manage the adverse effects of oral morphine: an evidence-based report. *J Clin Oncol,* 2001. 19: p. 2542-2554.

[164] Flores, C. and J. Mogil, The pharmacogenetics of analgesia: toward a genetially-based approach to pain management. *Pharmacogenomics,* 2001. 2: p. 177-194.

[165] Mogil, J., L. Yu, and A. Basbaum, Pain genes? natural variation and transgenic mutants. *Annu Rev Neurosci,* 2000. 23: p. 777-811.

[166] Pasternak, G., The pharmacology of mu analgesic: from patients to genes. *Neuroscientist,* 2001. 7: p. 220-231.

[167] Pan, X., et al., Identification and characterization of two new human mu opioid receptor splice variants hMOR-10 and hMOR-1X. *Biochem Biophys Res Commun,* 2003. 301: p. 1057-1061.

[168] Bolan, E. and G. Pasternak, Functional analysis of MOR-1 splice variants of the mu opioid receptor gene, Oprm. *Synapse,* 2004. 51: p. 11-18.

[169] Abbadie, C., X. Pan, and G. Pasternak, Differential distribution in rat brain of mu opioid receptor carboxy terminal splice variants MOR-1C and MOR-1 like immunoreactivity: evidence for region-specific processing. *J Comp Neurol,* 2000. 419: p. 244-256.

[170] Abbadie, C., et al., Comparative immunohistochemical distributions of carboxy terminus epitopes from the mu opioid receptor splice variants MOR-1D, MOR-1 and MOR-1C in the mouse and rat central nervous systems. *Neuroscience,* 2000. 100: p. 141-153.

[171] Abbadie, C., G. Pasternak, and S. Aicher, Presynaptic localization of the carboxy-terminus epitopes of the mu opioid receptor splice variants MOR-1C and MOR-1D in the superficial laminae of the rat spinal cord. *Neuroscience,* 2001. 106: p. 833-842.

[172] Brown, G., et al., 3-Methoxynaltrexone, a selective heroin/morphine-6Beta-glucuronide antagonist. *FEBS Lett,* 1997. 412: p. 35-38.

[173] Rossi, G., et al., Novel receptor mechanisms of heroin and morphine-6Beta-lucuronide analgesia. *Neurosci Lett,* 1996. 216: p. 1-4.

[174] Schuller, A., et al., Retention of heroin and morphine-6 beta-glucuronide analgesia in a new line of mice lacking exon 1 of MOR-1. *Nat Neurosci,* 1999. 2: p. 151-156.

[175] Walker, J., et al., Antagonism of heroin and morphine self-administration in rats by the morphine-6Beta-glucuronide antagonist 3-o-methylnaltrexone. *Eur J Clin Pharmacol,* 1999. 383: p. 115-119.

[176] Rossi, G., et al., Antisense mapping the MOR-1 opioid receptor: evidence for alternative splicing and a novel morphine-6Beta-glucuronide receptor. *FEBS Lett,* 1995. 369: p. 192-196.

[177] Rossi, G., K. Standifer, and G. Pasternak, Differential blockade of morphine and morphine-6Beta-glucuronide analgesia by antisense oligodeoxynucleotides directed against MOR-1 and G-protein alpha subunits in rats. *Neuroscie Lett,* 1995. 198: p. 99-102.

In Frontiers in Pain Research
Editor: Alexendre Lucas, pp.73-99

ISBN 1-59454-828-5

Chapter 4

THE PROMISE AND LIMITATIONS OF BROAD-SPECTRUM ANALGESICS: NICOTINIC ACETYLCHOLINE RECEPTOR AGONISTS AS A POTENTIAL CANDIDATE

Lynne E. Rueter, *** Prisca Honoré and R. Scott Bitner***
Abbott Laboratories, Neuroscience Research, Abbott Park, IL

ABSTRACT

Despite years of research and available medications, pain remains one of the most under-treated medical conditions. This is due, in part, to the complexity and heterogeneity of the condition itself. Both clinical and preclinical studies indicate that pain resulting from different etiologies develops and is maintained via differing biological processes. Pragmatically, this has culminated in the use of targeted analgesics, i.e. medications efficacious in and individually approved for only certain subtypes of pain. However, the desire to create non-opioid broad-spectrum analgesics remains as the treatment of pain would be greatly simplified if physicians did not have to tailor medication to each individual patient. Additionally, developing a broad-spectrum analgesic with an improved safety profile is paramount so that physicians and patients would not have to try to find the often inadequate but acceptable balance between moderate efficacy and tolerable side effects. Nicotinic acetylcholine receptor (nAChR) agonists have the potential to be broad-spectrum analgesics based on preclinical studies demonstrating efficacy in numerous pain states including multiple forms of acute, chronic, inflammatory and neuropathic pain. Intriguingly, research indicates that the exact mechanism(s) through which nAChR agonists induce analgesia may differ depending upon the type of pain, thus further supporting the contention that these compounds may have the appropriate biological properties to relieve a wide range of clinical pain states. However, given the ubiquitous distribution of nAChRs and the number of biological functions

* Corresponding author. e-mail: lynne.e.rueter@abbott.com; phone: 1-847-935-4292; fax: 1-847-938-0072

modulated by the nAChR system, achieving adequate pain relief without adverse side effects remains the greatest challenge. The present article will review the current understanding of pain states with regard to the development of broad-spectrum analgesics, using nAChR agonists as an example of the promise and challenges inherent in this approach.

BACKGROUND OF CLINICAL PAIN

The International Association for the Study of Pain (IASP) defines pain as an "unpleasant sensory and emotional experience associated with actual or potential tissue damage, or described in terms of such damage" (Merskey and Bugduk 1994). This definition clearly indicates that pain is a multidimensional experience. Pain is not homogenous and can be classified as acute or chronic. Acute or physiological pain is an early warning against potential injury, a vital defense mechanism, whereas chronic pain does not play any useful role. As such, chronic pain can be very detrimental to the individual's quality of life, disrupting sleep and normal living, and degrading health and functional capability (for review see Harden and Cohen 2003).

Chronic pain is one of the most common complaints for people soliciting medical help. It can affect general and psychological health (as is evident by the high degree of co-morbidity of chronic pain and emotional disorders such as depression and anxiety), and can also have deleterious socio-economic consequences since it is often associated with the loss of many work-days and an increased use of healthcare resources. Published estimates of the prevalence of chronic pain typically range from 2% to 45% (see Elliott et al, 1999 for references). In their epidemiology survey, Elliott et al (1999) published that 50.4% of the respondents reported suffering from chronic pain. Interestingly, there was no significant difference between sexes and, as could be expected, the proportion and the degree of pain significantly increased with age. Furthermore, Eriksen et al. (2003) showed that 33-40% of chronic pain patients included in their study were unhappy with medical examinations, medical tests, and treatments related to their chronic pain state. This lack of satisfactory pain relief in chronic pain patients was also identified in a 2004 "Americans living with Pain survey" done on behalf of the American Chronic Pain Association. In this study, 50% of the chronic pain patients surveyed felt that their pain was not under control. These alarming results clearly outline the need for better and more efficacious pain management medications, programs, and therapies. As will be discussed in detail below, one of the greatest challenges to creating more efficacious medications for pain control has been the heterogeneity of the condition itself including both the causes and underlying pathologies as well as the usefulness of current pharmacological therapies. One consistent desire in the field has been to develop a safe and tolerable broad-spectrum analgesic that would markedly simplify treatment programs, however, whether that is ultimately possible given the physiology of the condition remains to be determined.

Types of Clinical Chronic Pain

Chronic pain is defined as pain extending beyond the period of healing, and is usually not correlated with sufficient pathology that would explain the presence and/or extent of the pain. One exception would be progressive diseases such as cancer and arthritis where chronic pain is associated with demonstrable, often worsening, tissue damage. Chronic pain may be nociceptive, neuropathic, or both and can originate from cancer, injury, surgery, or chronic conditions such as arthritis or nerve injury/disease (for review see Jacobson and Mariano 2001, Turk and Okifuji 2001).

Chronic pain is usually divided further into cancer-related and chronic non-cancer pain. Cancer-related pain is a significant clinical problem that is likely to increase as the average life span of cancer patients continues to rise and cancer therapies continue to improve. It includes pain caused by the disease itself (tumor invasion of tissue, compression or infiltration of nerves or blood vessels, organ obstruction, infection, inflammation) and/or painful diagnostic procedures or treatments (biopsy, postoperative pain, chemotherapy or radiation therapy) (for review see Caraceni and Portenoy 1999, Portenoy and Lesage 1999). While cancer pain is considered to be a category of pain in itself, to date there is little published evidence to support a distinction between cancer-related and non-cancer-induced chronic pain based solely on underlying neural processes. Thus, in practice, clinicians discuss cancer-related pain in terms of acute or chronic pain, with underlining nociceptive and/or neuropathic components, as they would for non-cancer pain conditions.

As discussed above, the other subtype of chronic pain is chronic non-cancer pain. Typically, chronic non-cancer pain patients describe pain levels that are poorly correlated to the extent/presence of tissue injury/pathology and/or are not adequately relieved by standard analgesics. A main issue with chronic non-cancer pain is that it can persist for many years and can be of a wide variety of origins such as acute injury and various chronic conditions like osteoarthritis, low back pain, myofascial pain, fibromyalgia, headaches/migraines, central pain following spinal cord injury, stroke, or multiple sclerosis, chronic abdominal pain conditions such as ulcer or irritable bowel syndrome, phantom limb pain, peripheral neuropathy, and post-herpetic or trigeminal neuralgia. Chronic non-cancer pain can involve any region of the body, and the degree of pain can be anywhere from mild to unbearable. In addition, chronic non-cancer pain conditions also vary in terms of their characteristics. Some of them are easy to diagnose based on distinct characteristics, while some neuropathic pain conditions can be particularly difficult to identify, as they may exist without a known pathology (for review see Dunajcik 1999, Jacobson and Mariano 2001).

The Physiological Mechanisms of Pain

Both cancer-related and chronic non-cancer pain can be classified on the basis of their presumed underlying pathophysiology and are broadly categorized as nociceptive pain or neuropathic pain conditions. Nociceptive pain is caused by the ongoing activation of A-δ and C-nociceptors in response to a noxious stimulus (injury, disease, inflammation) (Figure 1). It can be further classified into visceral pain (deep cramping sensation associated with referred pain), superficial somatic pain (skin; well-localized sharp, pricking, or burning sensation), and deep somatic pain (muscle, joint capsules, and bone; diffuse dull or aching sensation).

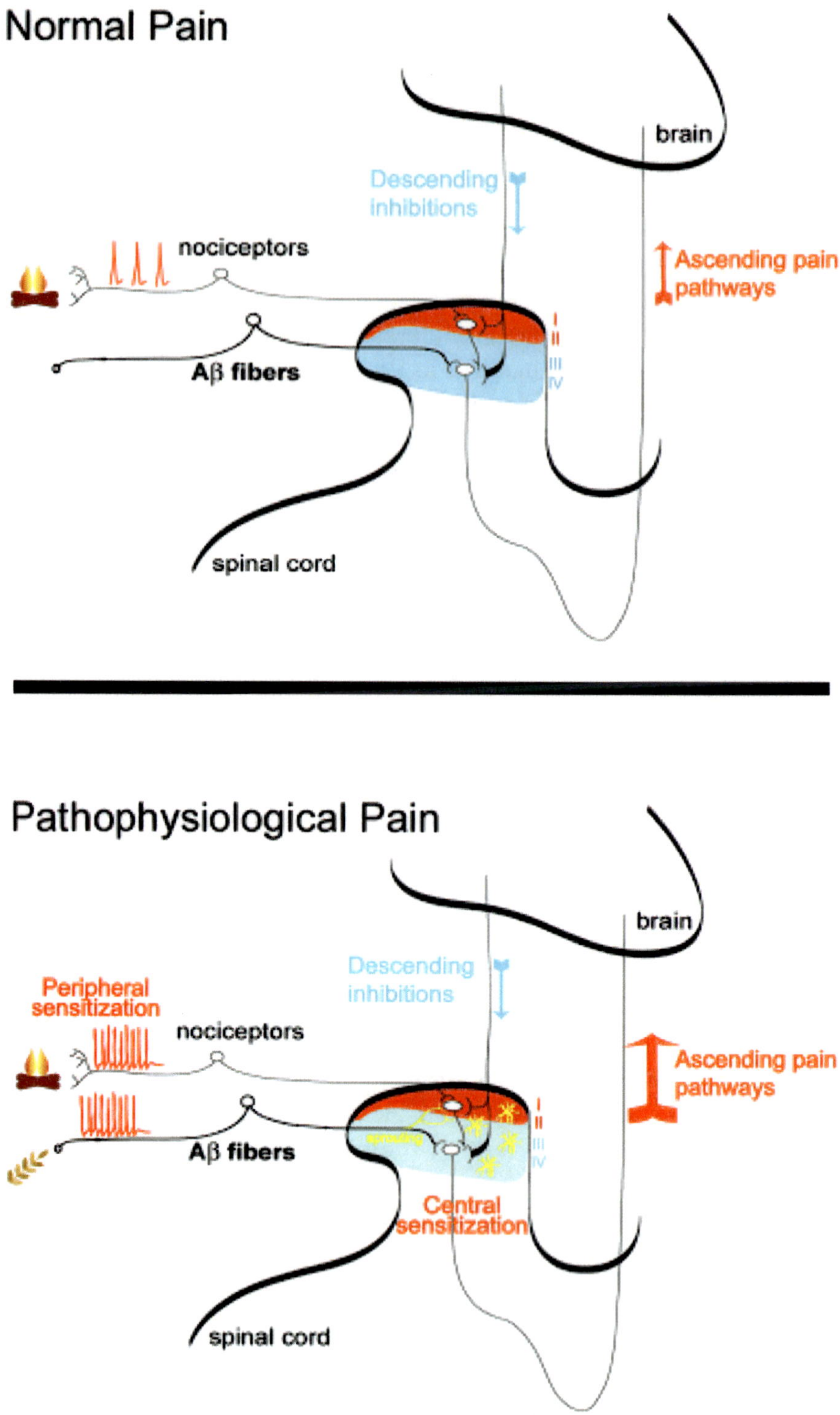

Figure 1. Normal and pathophysiological pain.

Usually, the nervous system associated with nociceptive pain is functioning properly, there is a close correspondence between pain perception and stimulus intensity, and the pain is indicative of real or potential tissue damage. As the system gets sensitized, in addition to spontaneous pain, nociceptive pain is also associated with evoked hyperalgesic and allodynic conditions (hyperalgesia: increased response to a painful stimulus; allodynia: pain caused by a normally innocuous stimulus) (for review see Coda and Bonica 2001, Byers and Bonica 2001, Meyer et al. 1985). In general, nociceptive pain abates completely upon the resolution of injury if the disease process is controlled. Because of this, the use of disease modifying therapies is being emphasized in the treatment of nociceptive chronic pain as illustrated in the treatment of rheumatoid arthritis not only by anti-inflammatory agents but also by biological therapies such as TNFα "antagonists" (Abbott and Moreland 2004).

Contrary to nociceptive pain, neuropathic pain can persist long after the initiating event has healed and is the expression of an abnormal processing of sensory information by the nervous system rather than a reaction to a pathology. Neuropathic pain can be classified as peripheral (painful peripheral mononeuropathy and polyneuropathy) or central (post stroke, following spinal cord injury) and can originate from nerve injury following a wide array of conditions/events such as direct trauma to nerves, inflammation/neuritis/nerve compression, metabolic diseases (diabetes), infections (herpes zoster, HIV), tumors (nerve compression/ infiltration), toxins (chemotherapy), and primary neurological diseases (for review see Backonja and Serra 2004a,b; Dworkin et al 2003; Smith 2004). Following nerve injury, changes occur in the CNS that can persist indefinitely. Under these conditions of sensitization, pain can occur without specific stimulus or can be disproportionate to the stimulus intensity. As for its characteristics, neuropathic pain may be constant or intermittent and is felt in many different ways (allodynia or hyperalgesia associated with mechanical or thermal stimuli but also spontaneous sensations such as burning, tingling, prickling, shooting, deep aching, and spasm) (for review see Backonja and Serra 2004a,b; Dworkin et al 2003; Smith 2004).

Sensitization

Two mechanisms play a key role in the development and maintenance of chronic pain, namely peripheral sensitization and central sensitization (Figure 1, Treede et al. 1992). Peripheral sensitization can result from the sensitization of nociceptors by inflammatory mediators (PGE2, 5-HT, bradykinin, epinephrine, adenosine), by neurotrophic factors released during tissue damage or by inflammatory cells, and also by intense, repeated, or prolonged noxious stimulation. Consequences of peripheral sensitization are a lowering of the activation threshold of nociceptors and an increase in their firing rate (Figure 1). These changes result in the production of hyperalgesia and allodynia associated with nociceptive chronic pain. In addition, peripheral sensitization also plays an important role in the development and maintenance of central sensitization (for review see Millan 1999; Woolf and Salter 2000).

Central sensitization (long-lasting increases in dorsal horn neuron excitability and responsiveness) is associated with spontaneous dorsal horn neuron activity, responses from neurons that normally only respond to low intensity stimuli (altered neural connections following sprouting of Aβ fibers to superficial laminae), expansion of dorsal horn neuron receptive fields, and reduction in central inhibition (Figure 1; Costigan and Woolf 2000, McMahon and Wall 1984, Woolf 1983, Woolf and Thompson 1991). Central sensitization is associated with persistent pain, hyperalgesia, allodynia, and the spread of pain to uninjured tissue, i.e. secondary hyperalgesia. In addition, it reflects a complex series of changes occurring in the spinal cord that may promote long-lasting increases in dorsal horn neuron excitability. While both peripheral and central sensitization play a role in nociceptive chronic pain, central sensitization clearly plays a key role in neuropathic pain. Thus, central sensitization also explains the observation that established pain is more difficult to suppress than acute pain because of the maladaptive changes that have taken place in the CNS (for review see Millan 1999; Woolf and Salter 2000). Interestingly, it has recently been shown that not only neurons, but also glial cells such as astrocytes and microglia are involved in the generation and maintenance of central sensitization (for review see Watkins et al 2001; Tsuda et al 2005).

Available Clinically Efficacious Pain Medications

Based on the diversity of the mechanisms underlining chronic pain (nociceptive/ neuropathic, various degrees of pain intensity, various ethiologies, peripheral/central sensitization, for review see Backonja and Serra 2004 a,b; Dickenson 1996; Millan 1999; Woolf and Salter 2000), all pain medications available to patients are not efficacious in all patients or in all pain conditions (Portenoy 2000). Analgesics can be broadly categorized as non-opioid analgesics (acetaminophen and non-steroidal anti-inflammatory drugs (NSAIDs)), opioid analgesics (morphine), and adjuvant analgesics or co-analgesics (antiepileptic drugs and antidepressants). In a simplistic classification, non-opioid analgesics are mostly used to relieve mild to moderate nociceptive pain, adjuvant analgesics are used to relieve neuropathic pain, and opioid analgesics are used to treat severe pain of all origins, depending on the dose prescribed.

The primary mechanism of action of NSAIDs is the blockade of prostaglandin synthesis through inhibition of the cyclo-oxygenase enzymes (COX-1 and COX-2). Non-opioid analgesics have anti-inflammatory, anti-pyretic, and analgesic effects, and their anti-inflammatory effects can indirectly relieve nociceptive pain by reducing inflammation and tissue swelling, although potency across these effects can be compound dependent. These characteristics make them particularly efficacious in nociceptive pain conditions associated with peripheral inflammation. Recently, selective inhibitors of COX-2, the COX enzyme isoform inducible by inflammation, have demonstrated the same efficacy with fewer GI side effects vs NSAIDs at therapeutic doses. However, they have recently been associated with a significant increase in the risk of cardiovascular disease (Davies and Jamali, 2004) which has brought the entire class under intense scrutiny. As stated above, non-opioid analgesics relieve mild to moderate pain associated with trauma, surgery, cancer, and arthritis. They are especially effective for certain types of somatic pain such as muscle and joint pain, sprains, bone/dental pain (tooth extraction), inflammatory pain, osteoarthritic pain, and in combination with disease modifying therapies in rheumatoid arthritic pain (for review see McCaffery and Portenoy 1999a,b, Hochberg 2002).

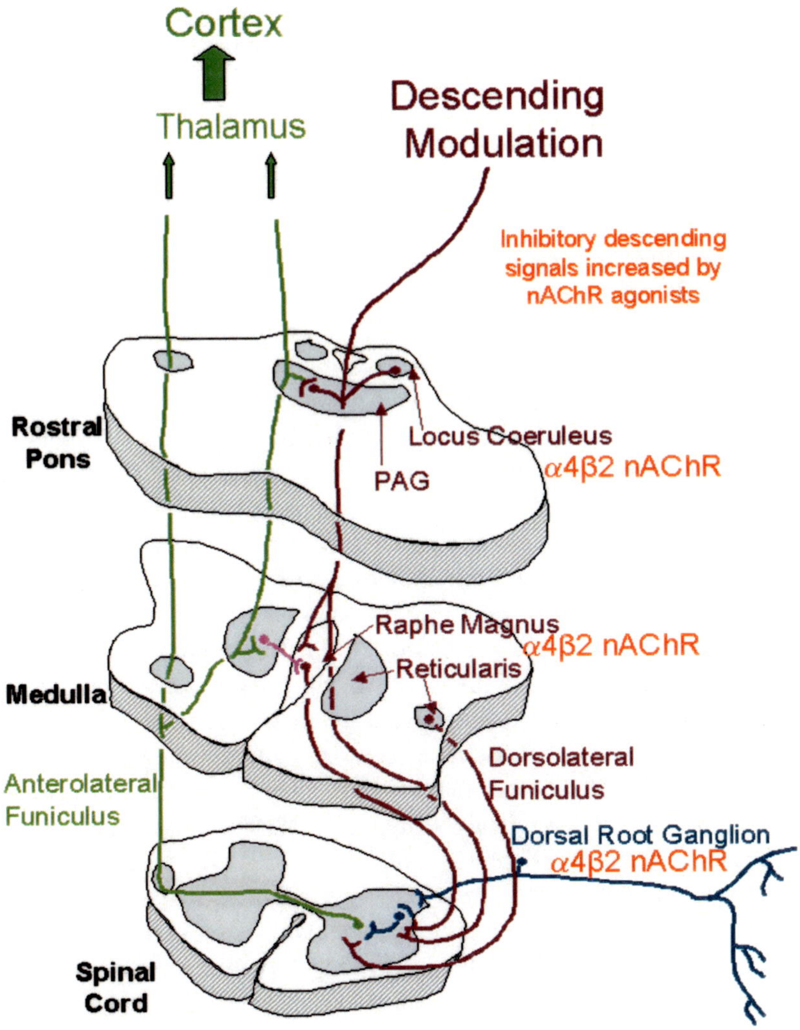

Figure 2. Major ascending and descending pathways involved in pain transmission and the location of nAChRs in the pathways.

Opioid analgesics produce their effects by binding and activating the opioid receptors in the CNS (for review see Pasero et al. 1999). Given the anatomical distribution of the opioid receptors in the CNS, opioid analgesics can block pain transmission from the periphery to the spinal cord by blocking neurotransmitter release from the primary afferent fibers and by directly decreasing activation of post-synaptic dorsal horn neurons. In addition, acting at higher brain centers, opioid analgesics can decrease pain transmission from the spinal cord to the brain, alter the limbic system, and increase descending inhibitory pathways to modulate pain transmission at the spinal level (see Figure 2). While nociceptive pain is generally more responsive to opioid analgesics than neuropathic pain, nearly all types of pain respond to the right dose of opioid analgesics. Opioid analgesics are usually recommended to treat moderate to severe pain that does not respond to non-opioid analgesics alone and are often prescribed in combination with non-opioid analgesics. They do play a key role in the treatment of acute pain (postoperative pain), breakthrough pain, cancer pain, and some types of chronic non-cancer pain (see Portenoy 2000, Portenoy and Lesage 1999). However, the use of opioid analgesics is associated with side effects such as sedation, confusion, respiratory depression, constipation, nausea and vomiting that can limit their utility as many patients cannot tolerate taking them.

The last class of analgesics used in the clinic is called adjuvant analgesics that have a primary indication other than pain but have demonstrated analgesic effects in particular pain conditions. Anti-epileptic drugs such as gabapentin and lamotrigine are a type of adjuvant analgesic and are used primarily in the treatment of neuropathic pain (for review see Backonja and Serra 2004a,b; McCleane 2003, 2004). While it is hypothesized that their analgesic effects are due to their ability to reduce membrane excitability and tone down a hyper-excitable nervous system, their exact mechanism(s) of action remain unclear and not all anti-epileptic drugs are good analgesics. As a class, they are most efficacious at treating peripheral neuropathic pain, post-herpetic neuralgia, trigeminal neuralgia, and diabetic neuropathic pain (for review see Hansson and Dickenson 2005). Recent data suggest that newer anti-epileptic drugs such as gabapentin or lamotrigine are better alternatives to older anti-epileptic drugs. Lamotrigine has been shown to be effective in patients with trigeminal neuralgia, complex regional pain syndrome, and neuropathic pain associated with multiple sclerosis and HIV (Backonja, 2002; Papagallo, 2003). In addition, it has been shown that gabapentin provides pain relief in diabetic neuropathic pain conditions and post-herpetic neuralgia; it also has a more favorable side effect profile compared to other neuropathic pain agents (Papagallo, 2003). Open label studies suggest that gabapentin also may be useful in the management of trigeminal neuralgia, central pain, phantom limb pain, and neuropathy associated with human immunodeficiency virus infection. Thus, many pain experts consider gabapentin a first-line treatment for neuropathic pain. Common side effects of anti-epileptic drugs as a class include sedation, mental clouding, dizziness, nausea, or unsteadiness, and patients need to start at low doses and go through a slow titration in order to diminish the risk of side effects. In addition to anti-epileptic drugs, tricyclic antidepressant drugs are also used as adjunct analgesics in the treatment of neuropathic pain (for review see Backonja and Serra 2004a,b; Dworkin et al 2003; McCleane 2003, 2004). While other antidepressant medications such as selective serotonin reuptake inhibitors have not proven to be particularly efficacious in treating neuropathic pain, some of the newer combination serotonin-norepinephrine reuptake inhibitors such as duloxetine and venlafaxine have been shown to significantly attenuate neuropathic pain (Briley, 2004). Indeed, duloxetine (Cymbalta) is one of the newest approved medication for the treatment of the pain associated with diabetic neuropathy (FDA Consum, 2004).

As discussed above, pain is a highly heterogeneous condition. There are multiple categories of pain including acute/physiological and chronic pain, cancer and non-cancer related pain, and nociceptive and neuropathic pain. In addition, pain can be of very diverse origins, including injury and disease as well as unknown etiologies. Finally, not all patients get pain relief, the presently available treatments differ based on the types of pain they effectively treat, and their use is greatly limited by side effects.

Given this diversity, whether a single non-opioid pharmacological approach could ever show broad-spectrum analgesia across a range of pain conditions has been brought into question. However, the possibility remains as does the desire to create a broad-spectrum analgesic that would simplify and improve the treatment of chronic pain. In order to suggest a single molecular mechanism as a possible safe broad-spectrum analgesic, it should meet several criteria including evidence for efficacy across multiple pain conditions, evidence for the ability to address differing underlying pathologies of pain, and evidence for an adequate safety window that will allow physicians to achieve analgesia in varying pain states. The remainder of this chapter will present nAChR agonists as possible candidates for broad-spectrum analgesics and will assess the degree to which they meet the criteria listed above.

Preclinical Animal Models of Pain

To study pain transmission, identify new pain targets, and characterize the potential analgesic profile of newly identified compounds designed for pain relief, an array of animal pain models has been developed mainly in rodents, reflecting all types of pain, from acute to chronic, somatic to visceral and nociceptive to neuropathic to cancer pain (Table 1). Depending on the model, pain measurements can encompass spontaneous pain behaviors (flinching, licking, biting, stretching) as well as evoked pain induced by a heat source (hot-plate, water bath, radiant heat), paw pressure (Randall Selitto), or tactile stimulation with von Frey monofilaments (force). Interestingly, the differential efficacy of the medications for different types of pain that is seen in the clinic is also observed when studying the effects of classical analgesic drugs in animal models of pain (Table 2). For example, while opioid analgesics like morphine are potent and efficacious in all animal models of pain, anti-inflammatory agents such as ibuprofen and celecoxib are most potent and effective in animal models associated with inflammation, and anti-epileptics like lamotrigine and gabapentin are most potent and efficacious in animal models of neuropathic pain (Table 2).

As preclinical models of the various forms of pain appear to have selective and differential predictive validity for efficacy in the clinical setting, they should be useful in determining if compounds with a novel molecular mechanism have the promise to be broad-spectrum analgesics. The next section will discuss the broad efficacy of nAChR agonists in preclinical models of acute nociceptive, chronic inflammatory and chronic neuropathic pain.

The Broad Spectrum Preclinical Profile of nAChR Agonists

The analgesic properties of nicotine have been recognized for many years (Davis et al, 1932); however, it was the isolation of epibatidine from the skin of the Ecuadoran tree frog *Epipedobates tricolor* in 1974 that sparked the investigation of nAChR agonists as a possible pharmacological treatment for pain (Daly et al, 2000). Since that time, nAChR agonists have been shown to be efficacious in a wide number of preclinical pain models believed to be representative of most clinical pain states. As importantly, they have been shown to be efficacious upon repeated administration, an aspect crucial to a potential clinically efficacious treatment (Bannon et al, 1998b,c). The specific preclinical pain models in which nAChR agonists have been assessed are discussed below as well as summarized in Table 1.

Table 1. Preclinical models of pain in rodents and effects of nAChR agonists.

Pain Type	Model	Description	Effect Demonstrating Analgesia	nAChR Agonists Showing Efficacy	References
Acute somatic	Tail flick	Focused light beam or Pinch	Increase latency (sec)	nicotine, epibatidine, ABT-594, SIB-1663, RJR 2403	Caggiula et al, 1995; Sullivan et al, 1996; Kesingland et al, 2000; Damaj et al, 1999; Rao et al, 2004
	Hot plate	Hot metal plate (50-55°C)	Increase latency to lick (sec)	nicotine, epibatidine, ABT-594, RJR 2403 and TC-2696	Caggiula et al, 1995; Sullivan et al, 1996; Bannon et al, 1998a; Damaj et al, 1999; Jordan et al, 2004
	Radiant heat	Focused light beam on plantar surface of hind paw	Increase paw withdrawal latency (sec)	ABT-594, A-85380, TC-2696	Bannon et al, 1998a; Rueter et al, 2000; Jordan et al, 2004
	Paw pressure	Compression of hind paw	Increase paw withdrawal threshold (g)	nicotine, RJR 2403	Damaj et al, 1999
	Formalin phase 1 (0-5 min)	Injection of formalin into one hind paw	Decrease number or duration of nocifensive behaviors	nicotine, RJR 2403	Damaj et al, 1999
Acute visceral	Abdominal constriction	Intraperitoneal injection of acetic acid or PPQ	Decrease number of constriction and stretching responses	epibatidine, ABT-594 and RJR 2403	Sullivan et al, 1996; Decker et al, 1998a; Damaj et al, 1999
Nociceptive somatic	Formalin phase 2 (20-60 min)	Injection of formalin into one hind paw	Decrease number or duration of nocifensive behaviors	nicotine, epibatidine, ABT-594, A-85380, RJR-2403 and BTG-102	Zarrindast et al, 2004; Sullivan et al, 1996; Bannon et al, 1998a; Curzon et al, 1998; Damaj et al, 1999; Hagan et al, 2003
	Skin incision	Incision of skin, fascia and muscle of hind paw	Increase paw withdrawal latency from heat, increase paw withdrawal threshold (force)	ABT-594	Gauvin et al, 2003
	Complete Freund's adjuvant (CFA)	Injection of CFA into one hind paw	Decrease inflammation, increase paw withdrawal latency from heat, increase paw withdrawal threshold from pressure	ABT-594, RJR-2403 and TC-2696	Kesingland et al, 2000; Damaj et al, 1999; Jordan et al, 2004

Table 1. Preclinical models of pain in rodents and effects of nAChR agonists. (Cont'd)

Pain Type	Model	Description	Effect Demonstrating Analgesia	nAChR Agonists Showing Efficacy	References
Neuropathic somatic	Spinal nerve ligation (SNL)	Tight ligation of L5-L6 spinal nerves	Increase paw withdrawal threshold (force)	ABT-594, A-85380 and nicotine	Bannon et al, 1998b; Kesingland et al, 2000; Rueter et al, 2003; Bannon et al, 1998b
	Sciatic nerve ligation (Chronic constriction injury)	Chronic loose constriction of the sciatic nerve	Increase paw withdrawal latency from heat, increase paw withdrawal threshold (force)	TC-2696	Jordan et al, 2004
	Partial sciatic nerve ligation	Tight ligation of 1/2 to 2/3 of the sciatic nerve	Increase paw withdrawal threshold (force)	ABT-594	Kesingland et al, 2000
	Diabetic neuropathy	Injection of streptozotocin	Increase paw withdrawal latency from pressure	ABT-594	Bannon et al, 1998b
	Chemotherapy	Vincristine infusion (i.v.)	Increase paw withdrawal threshold (force)	ABT-594	Lynch et al, 2005

Table 2. Effects of clinically used analgesics and ABT-594 in pre-clinical models of inflammatory and neuropathic pain. Degree of efficacy is denoted as follows: 0 = no efficacy; + = minimal efficacy; ++ = moderate/partial efficacy, +++ = good efficacy; ++++ = full and potent efficacy

	Inflammatory Pain	Neuropathic Pain	
	CFA[1]	SNL[2]	Vincristine
ABT-594	++++	++++	++++
Morphine	++++	++	++
Ibuprofen	++++	+	0
Celecoxib	+++	+	0
Gabapentin	++++	++++	+++
Lamotrigine	++	++++	+++

[1] Complete Freund's Adjuvant

[2] Spinal Nerve Ligation

Acute Nociceptive Pain

As described above, the most basic form of pain transmission is acute nociceptive pain. In preclinical settings, the most common acute pain assays investigate the effects of compounds on thermal pain. In the mouse hot plate assay, nAChR agonists including nicotine, epibatidine, ABT-594, RJR 2403 and TC-2696 induce antinociception (Caggiula et al, 1995; Sullivan et al, 1996; Bannon et al, 1998a; Damaj et al, 1999; Jordan et al, 2004).

Similarly, in rat assays of acute thermal pain such as tail flick and paw withdrawal, those same compounds, as well as A-85380 and SIB-1663, have been shown to have potent efficacy in increasing pain threshold (Caggiula et al, 1995; Sullivan et al, 1996; Kesingland et al, 2000; Bannon et al, 1998a; Damaj et al, 1999; Rueter et al, 2000; Rao et al, 2004).

Chronic Inflammatory Pain

Although nAChR agonists are active in preclinical models of acute thermal pain, this type of pain is not considered to be particularly important in terms of human clinical pain states. However, these compounds have shown similar efficacy and potency in animal models of inflammatory and persistent pain that are thought to replicate pathological inflammatory pain states in human. In the complete Freund's adjuvant (CFA) model of inflammatory pain, ABT-594, RJR-2403 and TC-2696 have been reported to have efficacy (Kesingland et al, 2000; Damaj et al, 1999; Jordan et al, 2004). Similarly, in the formalin model of persistent pain, the nAChR agonists nicotine, epibatidine, ABT-594, A-85380, RJR-2403 and BTG-102 can completely block the nociceptive behaviors of paw flinching and licking induced by intraplantar injections of formalin (Zarrindast et al, 2004; Sullivan et al, 1996; Bannon et al, 1998a; Curzon et al, 1998; Damaj et al, 1999; Hagan et al, 2003).

Chronic Non-Cancer and Cancer Neuropathic Pain

One of the most under-treated forms of clinical pain is neuropathic pain. As with acute and inflammatory pain, nAChR agonists also show efficacy in preclinical models of neuropathic pain. For example, ABT-594 can completely attenuate the mechanical allodynia and hyperalgesia associated with the spinal nerve ligation (SNL) and the partial sciatic nerve ligation models in the rat (Bannon et al, 1998b; Kesingland et al, 2000). A-85380 and nicotine have also shown efficacy in the SNL model (Rueter et al, 2003; Bannon et al, 1998b) while TC-2696 has been reported to reverse hyperalgesia associated with the chronic constriction injury model of neuropathic pain (Jordan et al, 2004). In addition to these models of specific nerve damage, ABT-594 reduces mechanical hyperalgesia in the streptozotocin-induced diabetic neuropathy model (Bannon et al, 1998b) and reduces mechanical allodynia in the vincristine model of chemotherapy-induced neuropathy (Lynch et al, 2005).

Other Forms of Pain

There are far more forms of clinically relevant pain than those encompassed in the inflammatory and neuropathic pain models listed above. Interestingly, nAChR agonists have been reported to be efficacious in quite a number of them. For example, epibatidine, ABT-594 and RJR 2403 show efficacy in the mouse abdominal constriction model of visceral pain (Sullivan et al, 1996; Decker et al, 1998a; Damaj et al, 1999). Furthermore, in a model of trigeminal pain, the formalin model of facial pain, epibatidine dose dependently reverses hyperalgesia (Gilbert et al, 2001). Finally, in the skin incision model of post-surgical pain,

ABT-594 reduces tactile allodynia and spontaneous pain associated with the skin damage (Gauvin et al, 2003).

This wide range of efficacy across preclinical models of varying forms of pain suggests that nAChR agonists hold the potential to be broad-spectrum analgesics in a clinical setting. As described below, the reason for their broad efficacy is likely due to the diversity of the nAChR system as well as the distribution pattern of nAChRs throughout the nervous system.

NACHR MOLECULAR STRUCTURE AND PHARMACOLOGY

The nicotinic acetylcholine receptor (nAChR) was originally named for its ability to respond to the plant alkaloid nicotine, in addition to acetycholine, when applied to various ex vivo ganglionic cell preparations (Dale, 1914). The subsequent discovery that nAChRs were also located on muscle endplates of the neuromuscular junction became, and still remains, one of the major areas of focus in the study of nAChRs (Fatt and Katz, 1952; Fertuck and Salpeter, 1974). However, in addition to the autonomic ganglia and neuromuscular junction, nAChRs are widely expressed throughout the mammalian central nervous system (CNS) where they are considered key for cholinergic-mediated fast synaptic transmission in response to endogenous acetylcholine, a major CNS neurotransmitter. Although the primary emphasis in studying cholinergic neurotransmission was initially placed on central muscarinic acetylcholine receptors, the molecular cloning of subunits that make up neuronal nAChRs has more recently placed efforts on elucidating the physiological and pharmacological implications of these receptors, including their role in modulating pain, as reviewed here.

Molecular Structure of Neuronal nAChRs

Neuronal nAChRs are pentameric ligand gated ion channels (LGICs) assembled from a family of subunit genes that, in contrast to the muscle nAChR, are composed of only α and β subunits. To date, the total number of mammalian neuronal nAChR subunits is eleven ($\alpha_{2\text{-}7}$, $\alpha_{9\text{-}10}$, $\beta_{2\text{-}4}$). Each subunit, approximately 500 amino acids in length, consists of four spanning transmembrane domains (M1-M4) with both the amino (N) and carboxyl (C) terminus located extracellularly. Both empirical techniques and secondary structure protein modeling have indicated that the nAChR ligand binding-recognition site represents an interface between the N terminals of two adjacent subunits, at least one of which must be an α subunit. Separate binding sites have also been described for non-competitive antagonists, non-competitive channel blocking antagonists, and allosteric modulators (Gotti and Clementi, 2004).

Pharmacological Classes of Neuronal nAChR

Neuronal nAChRs belong to a superfamily of LGICs that include $GABA_A$, glycine, and 5-HT_3 receptors and are commonly divided into two broad pharmacological classes defined by a high binding affinity, or lack thereof, for the snake toxin antagonist α-bungarotoxin (α-BTX). The α-BTX-insensitive nAChRs are composed of combinations of α and β subunits that bind agonists with nM affinity, whereas the α-BTX-sensitive nAChRs appear to consist of primarily α_7 homomers that bind agonists with μM affinity and α-BTX with nM affinity. As hetero-pentameric receptors, the α-BTX-insensitive nAChRs would seem to have the potential for a large number of native subunit-containing subtypes. However, functional expression of neuronal nAChRs in Xenopous oocytes and recombinant cell lines is only seen with certain subunit combinations. Both α_4 and α_3 can form functional "pairwise" combinations (α:β) with either β_2 or β_4, whereas α_5 and β_3 cannot (Chen and Patrick, 1997; Drisdel and Green, 2000).

Knowledge of the exact subunit combinations and stochiometries of native neuronal nAChRs is lacking, with only a few major subtypes recognized. In the brain, these include the $\alpha_4\beta_2$ combination, often referred to as the high affinity nicotine subtype (Flores et al, 1992), and the α-BTX-sensitive α_7 homomer (Seguela et al, 1993). In the autonomic ganglia, the $\alpha_3\beta_4$ pairwise combination is considered the predominant nAChR subtype, although a variety of α_3-containing combinations may exist including assemblage with α_5 and/or β_2 (Conroy and Berg, 1995; Flores et al, 1996).

Biophysical Properties of Neuronal nAChR

Pharmacological activation of nAChRs results in a conformational transition from a closed to open state, consistent with LGIC biophysics, that permits the exchange of cations, such as sodium, calcium and potassium, through the channel pore of the nAChR-containing cell. The α_7 nAChR subtype has a higher permeability to calcium and undergoes a more rapid agonist-induced desensitization in comparison to heteromeric, α-BTX-insensitive nAChRs (Seguela et al, 1993). However, because nAChRs have a high permeability for calcium, in particular the α_7 subtype, the rapid ionotropic signal generated by these receptors can be converted and sustained through multiple cellular signaling pathways, given the second-messenger properties of calcium (Dajas-Bailador and Wonnacott, 2004). To this extent, nAChRs may be coupled to modulatory phenomena that mediate medium- to long-term events involving various intracellular processes that underlie the diverse range of neuronal activities associated with nAChR pharmacology.

Location of nAChRs in the Pain Pathway

One of the aspects of the nAChR system that suggests that nAChR ligands have the potential to be broad-spectrum analgesics is the multiple locations of nAChRs throughout the pain pathway. Neuronal nAChRs are found on primary sensory neurons where nociceptive information is initiated in the periphery, in the cells body regions of these neurons, i.e. the dorsal root ganglion (DRG), the dorsal spinal cord where the first pain synapse is located, in the brainstem cell body regions that control descending innervation, as well as in the higher brain regions that integrate and perceive sensory information such as the thalamus and the cortex (Figure 2; Decker et al, 2004).

DIVERSITY OF NACHR MECHANISMS OF ANALGESIA

As stated above, nAChRs are expressed all along the pain pathway, thus they are in the position to alter pain transmission on many levels. Interestingly, research suggests that the manner in which the activation of nAChRs alters the expression of pain depends not only upon its anatomical location but, more intriguingly, upon the type of pain.

Acute Physiological Pain

Until quite recently, the majority of work performed in the effort to understand the mechanism of action of nAChR agonist-induced analgesia has used acute nociceptive models of thermal pain. A relatively consistent picture of both the site of action as well as the receptor subunits that mediate nAChR agonist-induced attenuation of acute thermal pain has emerged.

First, the site(s) of action of nAChR agonist-induced antinociception appear to be in the CNS, not in the peripheral nervous system (PNS). Antagonists such as chlorisondamine, a quaternary nAChR channel blocker that does not readily cross the blood brain barrier, have been used to demonstrate the central location. Thus, chlorisondamine given systemically where it will only block peripheral nAChR channels does not block antinociception induced by the systemic administration of nAChR agonists such as epibatidine and A-85380. In contrast, chlorisondamine given intracerebroventricularly (i.c.v.), where it will only block central nAChR channels completely blocks nAChR agonist-induced antinociception (Curzon et al, 1998).

The spinal cord plays a crucial role in the transmission of pain signals from the periphery to the brain centers where pain is ultimately perceived. nAChR subunits are prevalent in the spinal cord (Khan et al, 2003), however, studies investigating how activation of spinal nAChRs alters pain behaviors in the freely moving animal have led to inconsistent results. At lower concentrations in the rat, nAChR agonists such as A-85380, epibatidine and nicotine infused in the intrathecal space of the lumber region of the spinal cord induce pain-like behaviors as evidenced by spontaneous flinching of the hind paws and thermal hyperalgesia (Khan et al, 1998; Rueter et al, 2000). These observations are further supported by a recent report of an increase of the C-fiber reflex induced by the infusion of epibatidine into the spinal cord (Radek et al, 2004). In contrast, at higher concentrations, these compounds can induce a transient antinociception in the rat (Khan et al, 1998; Rueter et al, 2000). Interestingly, both the pronociceptive and antinociceptive effects can be blocked by pretreatment with nonselective nAChR antagonists, but they are differentially antagonized by subunit selective antagonists (Khan et al, 1998; Rueter et al, 2000). However, the higher concentrations infused in these experiments are unlikely to be achieved following systemic administration of a nAChR agonist, which brings into question the physiological relevance of the antinociceptive findings and suggests that the central site of action of nAChR agonist-induced antinociception in acute thermal pain models is not at the level of the spinal cord. Interestingly, the intrathecal administration of nAChR agonists in the mouse has not been reported to induce pronociceptive behaviors but rather has been reported to lead to a far more consistent induction of antinociception in models such as the hot plate assay (Damaj et al

1998). However, the concentrations infused in those studies are also high enough to bring into question their physiological relevance.

While the evidence for the activation of nAChR at the level of the spinal cord being the mechanism by which systemically administered nAChR agonists induce antinociception in acute pain models is not consistent, the theory that pain signaling in the spinal cord is altered via nAChR-mediated alteration of descending inhibition is supported by convergent evidence from multiple sources. The antinociceptive actions of systemically administered nAChR agonists such as nicotine and A-85380 can be attenuated by the infusion of muscarinic, noradrenergic and serotonergic antagonists into the spinal cord (Iwamoto, 1989; Rueter et al, 2000). In addition, A-85380 has been demonstrated to increase the release of 5-HT in the lumbar spinal cord (Rueter et al, 2000). The site of action for nAChR agonists in the descending inhibition mediated by the serotonergic, noradrenergic and muscarinic system can be traced to the brainstem cell body regions of these neurons. First, at antinociceptive doses, agonists such as ABT-594 strongly activate the nucleus raphe magnus (NRM) and the locus coeruleus (LC), the cell body regions of descending serotonergic and noradrenergic neurons, respectively, as demonstrated by increased c-fos expression (Bitner et al, 1997, 1998). Second, infusion of nAChR agonists directly into the NRM can induce antinociception in an acute thermal pain model in the rat (Iwamato, 1989; Curzon et al, 1998). Third, deactivation of the NRM with lidocaine or destruction of the NRM using a neurochemical lesion can block antinociception induced by some nAChR agonists (Curzon et al, 1998; Decker et al, 1998b). Fourth, infusion of epibatidine into the NRM decreases the spinal C fiber reflex (Radek et al, 2004). Finally, infusion of nicotine into the mesopontine tegmentum, which contains the cell bodies of descending cholinergic neurons induces antinociception in acute thermal pain models (Iwamoto, 1989,1991). Together, these data strongly support a supraspinal location of nAChR agonist-mediated antinociception in acute pain that alters pain perception, at least in part, by enhancing descending inhibitory control of spinal cord activation.

One of the final pieces of the puzzle regarding the mediation of acute thermal pain by nAChR agonists involves the determination of the specific subunits responsible for these actions. By and large, evidence supports the importance of the $\alpha_4\beta_2$ subunit combination in nAChR agonist induced antinociception. First, the α_4 and β_2 preferential competitive antagonist dihydro-β-erythroidine (DHβE) can block antinociception induced by nAChR agonists (Damaj et al, 1998). Second, nicotine fails to induce antinociception in the hot-plate assay of acute thermal pain in mice lacking the α_4 receptor subunit and induces a very limited antinociception in mice lacking the β_2 receptor subunit (Marubio et al, 1999). Interestingly, in keeping with the supraspinal mediation discussed in the previous paragraph, NRM neurons in these knockout mice are no longer sensitive to nicotine-induced activation (Marubio et al, 1999). Third, selective knockdown of the α_4 receptor subunit using antisense markedly attenuates the antinociceptive effects of A-85380 (Bitner et al, 2000). While the role of other nAChR subunits such as the α_3 or the α_7 subunit have been suggested (Plenge et al, 2002; Damaj et al, 2000), the experimental evidence most consistently supports the $\alpha_4\beta_2$ subunit combination as being the most important for nAChR agonist-induced antinociception in acute thermal pain.

While the majority of work using acute thermal pain assays indicate a central site of action for nAChR agonist-induced antinociception, there is one interestingly consistent outlier. In the tail flick assay, an assay believed to be mediated predominately by spinal reflexes instead of supraspinal circuits, there appears to be both a peripherally mediated as well as a non-$\alpha_4\beta_2$ component to nAChR agonist induced efficacy. For example, unlike the paw withdrawal assay, quaternary compounds that do not readily cross the blood-brain barrier, e.g. hexamethonium, can block nicotine-induced antinociception in the tail flick assay (Caggiula et al, 1995). In addition, unlike the hot-plate assay, nicotine is still capable of inducing full analgesia in the tail flick assay in both α_4 and β_2 knockout mice, although it does require a significantly higher dose of nicotine (Marubio et al, 1999). These model and/or pain-dependent differences in nAChR agonist alleviation of pain will become even more apparent in the next section.

Chronic Neuropathic Pain

Recent research in the nAChR field has spent more effort in attempting to define the mechanism(s) of action of agonists in more clinically relevant forms of pain including chronic and neuropathic pain. While there are some similarities to acute pain, it is the mechanisms that appear to be specific to neuropathic pain that suggest nAChR agonists may hold unique potential as a broad-spectrum analgesic.

As stated above, nAChR agonist-induced antinociception in acute pain appears to be predominately centrally mediated, mainly in supraspinal cell body regions that alter pain transmission via descending inhibition into the spinal cord. In contrast, the analgesic actions of nAChR agonists in models of neuropathic pain appear to be mediated at multiple sites throughout the pain pathway. In particular, evidence suggests that there is an important peripheral component to nAChR agonist-induced anti-allodynia. In the SNL model of neuropathic pain, agonists such as ABT-594 and A-85380 fully block mechanical allodynia following systemic administration (Bannon et al, 1998b; Rueter et al, 2003). Interestingly, this anti-allodynic action can be completely antagonized by either central infusion or by systemic pretreatment with chlorisondamine, a quaternary nAChR channel blocker that does not readily cross the blood-brain barrier (Rueter et al, 2003). A peripheral site of action for nAChR agonists in neuropathic pain is further supported by a recent report that showed peripherally administered chlorisondamine was also able to partially attenuate ABT-594-induced anti-allodynia in the vincristine model of chemotherapy induced neuropathy (Lynch et al, 2005). Interestingly, the ability of peripherally administered chlorisondamine to attenuate nAChR agonist-induced anti-allodynia is much greater in the SNL model than in the vincristine model, suggesting there may even be diversity of pain mechanisms within neuropathies resulting from different etiologies.

To date, evidence suggests that the peripheral site of action is unlikely to be the primary receptive field as injections of small, site-specific doses of A-85380 directly into the paw do not attenuate SNL-induced allodynia (Rueter et al, 2003). In contrast, transient but complete anti-allodynia can be achieved by infusing nAChR agonists into the region of the injured DRG (Rueter et al, 2003). The idea that the DRG may play a different role in neuropathic pain than in acute pain is supported by changes induced in the DRG by these preclinical models. Peripheral axotomy of the sciatic nerve leads to upregulation of some nAChR subunits (Xiao et al, 2002). Indeed, changes in the degree to which DRG neurons acutely dissected from SNL rats are responsive to nAChR agonists have been observed. Interestingly, agonist-induced responses are drastically reduced, not increased as the behavioral or gene expression data might have predicted (Dubé et al, 2005). Thus, neuropathic pain models have been shown to change the configuration and properties of nAChRs in the DRG, however, the exact mechanism through which nAChR agonists attenuate pain at the level of the DRG remains to be understood.

Similar to the difference between acute and neuropathic pain states in terms of a peripheral site of action for nAChR agonists, the spinal cord also appears to be a more relevant site of action in neuropathic pain than in acute pain. Whereas intrathecal administration of nicotine or epibatidine does not alter mechanical pain threshold in normal mice, both agonists have been shown to be anti-allodynic following intrathecal administration in the partial sciatic nerve model (Rashid and Ueda, 2002). Again, a specific role for nAChR agonists in neuropathic pain at the level of the spinal cord is supported by gene changes seen in the spinal cord following nerve injury models such as axotomy of the sciatic nerve (Yang et al, 2004). Multiple nAChR subunits, including the α_5 and β_2 subunits, have been shown to be upregulated following surgery (Yang et al, 2004).

The subunits underlying the analgesic action in neuropathic pain models are less well defined than those involved in acute pain models. To date, a novel role for the α_5 subunit has been suggested by the ability of α_5 antisense to alleviate mechanical allodynia induced in the SNL model (Vincler and Eisenach, 2005). As the investigation of the mechanisms of nAChR agonists in neuropathic pain models is actually relatively new, quite a bit remains unknown.

One of the greatest challenges to creating a broad-spectrum analgesic has been the diversity of pain conditions in the clinic and their mediation by peripheral and central sensitization. It appears that nAChR agonists hold the promise to be broad-spectrum analgesics based on their activity in a wide range of preclinical models of pain, their ubiquitous location throughout the pain pathway, and their differential mediation of analgesia in different pain states. However, it is their wide distribution throughout the central and peripheral nervous system that has been the greatest challenge in bringing forth a clinical candidate.

Separating nAChR-Mediated Analgesia from Adverse Liabilities

The wide distribution of nAChRs within and outside the CNS and the diverse molecular makeup of subtypes, while likely an integral component to the broad-spectrum analgesic profile associated with nicotinic agonists, may contribute to a variety of adverse and undesirable effects. Stimulation or blockade of nAChRs located on parasympathetic and sympathetic post-ganglionic neurons can lead to the disruption of autonomic homeostasis, particularly in the urinary, cardiovascular, and gastrointestinal systems (Decker et al, 2004). Central nAChR activation is linked to a variety of side effects observed in preclinical animal testing. Moreover, neuronal nAChRs mediate the addictive properties of nicotine associated with cigarette smoking. Finally, alteration of nicotinic cholinergic transmission at the neuromuscular junction, such as respiratory muscles of the diaphragm, can also have adverse consequences. Therefore, a key issue in the consideration of this novel class of analgesic agents is to what extent, if any, the analgesia can be separated from potential side effect liabilities.

Separating Ganglionic nAChR-Mediated Liabilities

Both pharmacological and genetic strategies have been employed in trying to elucidate the side effect profile observed with pharmacological activation of nAChRs, particularly with respect to the adverse effects associated with the autonomic functioning, that are likely mediated through the $\alpha_3\beta_4$ subtype (Flores et al, 1996). Indeed α_3 and β_4 knockout mice display a phenotype consistent with autonomic dysfunction involving the gastrointestinal, urinary, and cardiovascular systems (Wang et al, 2002). However, whether nicotinic analgesics lacking α_3 activity would still demonstrate full antinociceptive activity is unknown. Reduced acute thermal pain observed in rats following direct injections of epibatidine into the medial habenula, a dense α_3 -expressing region of the thalamus that retains epibatidine autoradiographic binding in α_4 and β_2, but not in α_3, knockout mice, may suggest a possible antinociceptive role for the α_3 subunit in the brain (Plenge et al, 2002; Whiteaker et al, 2002).

Interestingly, it has also been suggested that activation of ganglionic nAChRs could play a role in analgesia. It has been speculated that pressor effects may indirectly mediate the antinociceptive effects of nicotine (Jamner et al, 1998). Baroreceptor stimulation can diminish the sensation of pain in smokers, but this appears to be dependent on smoking history. It has also been demonstrated that increasing baroreceptor stimulation using a neck cuff reduced pain perception in heavy smokers but not in nonsmokers or smokers who smoked fewer than 20 cigarettes per day (Rau et al, 1993). Moreover, the antinociceptive effects of the nAChR agonist ABT-594 are observed in rats at doses that do not increase blood pressure. Thus, it appears that indirect effects mediated by activation of the cardiovascular system cannot completely account for the analgesic effects of nAChR activation.

Separating CNS nAChR-Mediated Liabilities

Studies demonstrating reduced nicotinic antinociception in knockout mice (Marubio et al, 1999) or antisense-treated rats (Bitner et al, 2000) targeting the α_4 or β_2 subunit suggest that nAChR-mediated antinociception is through the $\alpha_4\beta_2$ subtype. Thus, $\alpha_4\beta_2$ selective agonists may be capable of producing analgesia devoid of autonomic side effects. However, the $\alpha_4\beta_2$ subtype itself may be responsible for some of the undesirable effects associated with nicotinic compounds. Decreased nicotine intravenous self-administration has been observed in β_2 knockout mice, suggesting that the $\alpha_4\beta_2$ subtype may contribute to nicotine abuse liability (Picciotto et al, 1998). Other side effects associated with pharmacological activation of central nAChRs include: hypothermia (Damaj et al, 1996), hyperlocomotion and excitation (Leikola-Pelho and Jackson, 1992) hypolocomotion and sedation (Clarke and Kumar, 1983), emesis (Beleslin and Krstic, 1987), and seizures (Damaj et al, 1999). Although the $\alpha_4\beta_2$ subtype is regarded as the predominant nicotinic subtype in the brain, some of these adverse effects are still present in mutant α_4 and β_2 knockout mice (Marubio et al, 1999), suggesting that other CNS subtypes, such as α_3-containing neuronal nAChRs (Adams et al, 2004) may be involved in mediating nicotinic-related liabilities.

From a clinical standpoint, the abuse potential of novel broad-spectrum analgesics will likely be a major consideration since opioids, well known for addiction liabilities and abuse, are currently the only broad-spectrum class of analgesics. Interestingly, in preclinical assays, nAChR agonists do not show an opioid-like abuse potential. For example, discontinuation of morphine following repeated dosing in rats produces decreased food intake, a measure of withdrawal and physical dependence, but when discontinuing a similar repeated dosing regimen of the nicotinic agonist ABT-594, food intake immediately returns to control levels (Bannon et al, 1998a). In other studies, Bannon and colleagues (1998a) also reported that ABT-594, in contrast to morphine, did not serve as a reinforcer in rats in the place preference test. Together, these results suggest that ABT-594 does not share the abuse profile of morphine in preclinical models.

Although nAChR agonists are unlikely to have the potential for opiate-like abuse, it is important to address the possibility of subtype selective nAChR agonists demonstrating a nicotine-like abuse potential. Studies in knockout mice indicate that nicotine intravenous self-administration is likely mediated through β_2-containing nAChRs (Picciotto et al, 1998). However, any potential abuse liability will likely be markedly limited by method and rate of administration. For example, inhalation through cigarette smoking achieves very rapid and high brain levels of nicotine likely optimal for the development of addiction (Slade and Henningfield, 1998). In contrast, slower and more continuous delivery of nicotine, such as transdermal patches, has significantly lower abuse potential (Pickworth et al, 1994). This contention is further supported by preclinical work that shows self-administration in rodents is obtainable predominately when nicotine is given intravenously, a method that mirrors the very rapid and high brain levels of nicotine seen during cigarette smoking. Therefore, the potential abuse liability of a novel nicotinic analgesic is likely to be influenced not only by pharmacodynamic properties, such as receptor subtype selectivity, but also pharmacokinetic properties and perhaps more importantly the drug delivery system used for administration.

Separating Neuromuscular nAChR-Mediated Liabilities

Effects on neuromuscular nAChRs can also lead to adverse consequences. Continuous pharmacological activation of neuromuscular nAChRs may lead to depolarization blockade, and in the case of muscles of the diaphragm, result in respiratory paralysis. This is certainly a concern for agonists with high affinity for neuromuscular nAChRs, such as epibatidine, which does produce respiratory depression. However, agonists with low affinity for neuromuscular nAChRs, such as ABT-594, probably do not present this liability, as effects on the respiratory system are significantly reduced in this compound (Decker et al, 1998b; Boyce et al, 2000). This again suggests the pharmacological ability to separate side effects from efficacious activity of nicotinic compounds.

Together, these data suggest that a nAChR agonist efficacious against multiple forms of clinically relevant pain with a reduced side effect profile is achievable. By targeting specific subunit combinations, most autonomic and neuromuscular liabilities could be avoided. In addition, many of the CNS-mediated side effects such as seizures and emesis could be markedly reduced.

SUMMARY AND CONCLUSIONS

Pain is a complex and heterogeneous state that continues to be one of the most under-treated medical conditions. Divided into various classes including acute physiological and chronic cancer- and non-cancer related nociceptive and neuropathic pain, the treatment for clinical pain remains limited. Interestingly, similar to the physiological differences underlying varying pain states, different classes of medications have proven to be useful for each of these states. However, each class of medications is limited either by degree of efficacy or by marked side effects that restrict their usefulness. Physicians must attempt to tailor and titrate the pharmacological treatment of pain to each individual patient, often failing to adequately relieve pain because of the limited efficacy of available medications, the occurrence of intolerable side effects, the inability to understand the true state of the patient and/or the fear of addiction to opioids. Thus, the medical and research community has desired to create a broad-spectrum analgesic with good efficacy and good tolerability that could simplify and improve the treatment of chronic pain. However, given the heterogeneity of pain, it has been questioned whether a broad-spectrum analgesic is possible.

Neuronal nAChR agonists hold the promise to be broad-spectrum analgesics. They are active in a wide range of preclinical pain models that have been shown to have predictive validity for activity in chronic nociceptive and neuropathic pain states. In addition, the mechanism(s) by which nAChR agonists induce analgesia are dependent upon the pain state. The analgesic efficacy has predominately been traced to one subunit combination, i.e. the $\alpha_4\beta_2$ subunit combination, thereby suggesting that potential cardiovascular, gastrointestinal, and respiratory side effects shown to be mediated by other subunit combinations could be avoided. Thus, the preclinical rationale for broad-spectrum efficacy with reduced side effects for subtype selective nAChR agonists is strong. It remains to be determined if this profile will translate to clinical efficacy.

REFERENCES

Abbott JD; Moreland LW. Rheumatoid arthritis: developing pharmacological therapies. *Exp Opin Investig Drugs*, 2004 13, 1007-1018.

Adams, MR; Nikkel, AL; Donnelly-Roberts, DL; Watt, AT; Johnston, JF; Cowsert ,LM; Butler, M; Kroeger, PE; Frost, L; Curzon, P; Decker, MW; Bitner, RS. In vitro and in vivo effects of an alpha3 neuronal nicotinic acetylcholine receptor antisense oligonucleotide. *Brain Res Mol Brain Res*, 2004 129, 67-79.

Backonja, M-M. Use of anticonvulsants for treatment of neuropathic pain. *Neurology*. 2002, 59, S14-17.

Backonja, M-M; Serra, J. Pharmacologic management part 1: better-studied neuropathic pain diseases. *Pain Medicine*, 2004a 5, S28-S47.

Backonja, M-M; Serra, J. Pharmacologic management part 2: lesser-studied neuropathic pain diseases. *Pain Medicine* 2004b 5, S48-S59.

Bannon, AW; Decker, MW; Holladay, MW; Curzon, P; Donnelly-Roberts, D; Puttfarcken, PS; Bitner, RS; Diaz, A; Dickenson, AH; Porsolt, RD; Williams, M; Arneric, SP. Broad-spectrum, non-opioid analgesic activity by selective modulation of neuronal nicotinic acetylcholine receptors. *Science* 1998a, 279, 77-81.

Bannon, AW; Decker, MW; Kim, DJB; Campbell, JE; Arneric, SP. ABT-594, a novel cholinergic channel modulator, is efficacious in nerve ligation and diabetic neuropathy models of neuropathic pain. *Brain Res* 1998b, 801, 158-163.

Bannon, AW; Decker, MW; Curzon, P; Buckley, MJ; Kim, DJB; Radek, RJ; Lynch, JK; Wasicak, JT; Lin NH; Arnold, WH; Holladay, MW; Arneric, SP. ABT-594 [5-((2R)-azetidinylmethozy)-2-chloropryridine]: a novel, orally effective antinociceptive agent acting via neuronal nicotinic acetylcholine receptors: II. in vivo characterization. *J Pharmacol Exp Ther* 1998c, 285, 787-794

Beleslin, DB; Krstic, SK. Further studies on nicotine-induced emesis: nicotinic mediation in area postrema. *Physiol Behav* 1987, 39, 681-686.

Bitner, RS; Nikkel, AL; Curzon, P; Arneric, SP; Bannon, AW; Decker, MW. Role of the nucleus raphe magnus in antinociception produced by ABT-594: immediate early gene responses possibly linked to neuronal nicotinic acetylcholine receptors on serotonergic neurons. *J Neurosci* 1998, 18, 5426-5432.

Bitner, RS; Nikkel, AL; Curzon, P; Donnelly-Roberts, DL; Puttfarcken, PS; Namovic, M; Jacobs, IC; Meyer, MD; Decker, MW. Reduced nicotinic receptor-mediated antinociception following in vivo antisense knock-down in rat. *Brain Res* 2000, 871, 66-74.

Bitner, RS; Nikkel, AL; Bannon, AW; Arneric, SP; Decker, MW. Supraspinal c-fos induction produced by a novel cholinergic channel modulator analgesic, ABT-594. *Soc Neurosci Abstr* 1997, 23, 1200.

Boyce, S; Webb, JK; Shepheard, SL; Russell, MGN; Hill, RG; Rupniak, NMJ: Analgesic and toxic effects of ABT-594 resemble epibatidine and nicotine in rats. *Pain* 2000, 85, 443-450.

Briley, M. Clinical experience with dual action antidepressants in different chronic pain syndromes. *Hum Psychopharmacol* 2004,19 Suppl 1, S21-25.

Byers, M; Bonica, JJ. Peripheral pain mechanisms and nociceptor plasticity. In: Loeser JD, Butler SH, Chapman CR, editors. *Bonica's Management of Pain. 3rd edition*. Baltimore, MD: Lippincott Williams & Wilkin; 2001; 26-72.

Caggiula, AR; Epstein, LH; Perkins, KA; Saylor, S. Different methods for assessing nicotine-induced antinociception may engage different neural mechanisms. *Psychopharmacology* 1995, 122, 301-306.

Caraceni, A; Portenoy, RK. An international survey of cancer pain characteristics and syndromes. IASP Task Force on Cancer Pain. International Association for the Study of Pain. *Pain* 1999, 82, 263-74.

Chen, DN; Patrick, JW. The alpha-bungarotoxin-binding nicotinic acetylcholine-receptor from rat-brain contains only the alpha-7 subunit. *J Biol Chem* 1997, 272, 24024-24029.

Clarke, PB; Kumar, R. The effects of nicotine on locomotor activity in non-tolerant and tolerant rats. *Br J Pharmacol* 1983, 78, 329-337.

Coda, BA; Bonica, JJ. General considerations of acute pain. In: Loeser, JD; Butler, SH; Chapman, CR, editors. *Bonica's Management of Pain. 3rd edition*. Baltimore, MD: Lippincott Williams & Wilkins; 2001; 222-240.

Conroy, WG; Berg, DK. Neurons can maintain multiple classes of nicotinic acetylcholine receptors distinguished by different subunit compositions. *J Biol Chem* 1995, 270, 4424-4431.

Costigan, M; Woolf, CJ. Pain: molecular mechanisms. *J Pain* 2000, 1, 35-44.

Curzon, P; Nikkel, AL; Bannon, AW; Arneric, SP; Decker, MW. Differences between the antinociceptive effects of the cholinergic channel activators A-85380 and (+/-)-epibatidine in rats. *J Pharmacol Exp Ther* 1998, 287, 847-853.

Dajas-Bailador, F; Wonnacott, S. Nicotinic acetylcholine receptors and the regulation of neuronal signalling. *Trends Pharmacol Sci* 2004, 25, 317-324.

Dale HH. The action of certain esters and ethers of choline, and their relation to muscarine. *J Pharmacol Exp Ther* 1914, 6, 147-190.

Daly, JW; Garraffo, HM; Spande, TF; Decker, MW; Sullivan, JP; Wiliams, M. Alkaloids from frog skin: the discovery of epibatidine and the potential for developing novel non-opioid analgesics. *Nat Prod Rep* 2000, 17, 131-135.

Damaj, MI; Fei-yin, M; Dukat, M; Glassco, W; Glennon, RA; Martin, BR. Antinociceptive responses to nicotinic acetylcholine receptor ligands after systemic and intrathecal administration in mice. *J Pharmacol Exp Ther* 1998, 284, 1058-1065.

Damaj, MI; Glassco, W; Aceto, MD; Martin, BR. Antinociceptive and pharmacological effects of metanicotine, a selective nicotinic agonist. *J Pharmacol Exp Ther* 1999, 291, 390-398.

Damaj, MI; Welch, SP; Martin, BR. Characterization and modulation of acute tolerance to nicotine in mice. *J Pharmacol Exp Ther* 1996, 277, 454-461.

Damaj, MI; Meyer, EM; Martin, BR. The antinociceptive effects of alpha 7 nicotinic agonists in an acute pain model. *Neuropharmacology* 2000, 39, 2785-2791.

Davies, NM; Jamali, F. COX-2 selective inhibitors cardiac toxicity: getting to the heart of the matter. *J Pharm Pharm Sci* 2004, 7, 332-336.

Davis, L; Pollock, LJ; Stone, T. Visceral pain. *Surg Gynecol Obstet* 1932, 55, 418-426.

Decker, MW; Bannon, AW; Buckley, MJ; Kim, DJB; Holladay, MW; Ryther, KB; Lin, NH; Wasicak, JT; Williams, M; Arneric. SP. Antinociceptive effects of the novel neuronal nicotinic acetylcholine receptor agonist, ABT-594, in mice. *Eur J Pharmacol* 1998a, 346, 23-33.

Decker, MW; Curzon, P; Holladay, MW; Nikkel, AL; Bitner, RS; Bannon, AW;, Donnelly-Roberts, DL; Puttfarcken, PS; Kuntzweiler, TA; Briggs, CA; WIlliams, M; Arneric, SP. The role of neuronal nicotinic acetylcholine receptors in antinociception: effects of ABT-594. *J Physiol* 1998b, 92, 221-224.

Decker, MW; Rueter, LE; Bitner RS. Nicotinic acetylcholine receptor agonists: a potential new class of analgesics. *Curr Top Med Chem 4*, 2004, 369-384.

Dickenson, AH. Balances between excitatory and inhibitory events in the spinal cord and chronic pain. *Prog Brain Res* 1996, 110, 225-231.

Drisdel, RC; Green, WN. Neuronal alpha-bungarotoxin receptors are alpha7 subunit homomers. *J Neurosci* 2000, 20, 133-139.

Dubé, GR, Kohlhaas, KL; Rueter, LE; Surowy, CS; Meyer, MD; Briggs, CA. Loss of functional neuronal nicotinic receptors in dorsal root ganglion neurons in a rat model of neuropathic pain. *Neurosci Lett* 2005, 376, 29-34.

Dunajcik L. Chronic nonmalignant pain. In: McCaffery, M; Pasero, C, editors. *Pain Clinical Manual, 2nd edition.* St. Louis, MO: Mosby Inc; 1999; 467-521.

Dworkin, RH; Backonja, M; Rowbotham, MC; Allen, RR; Argoff, CR; Bennett, GJ; Bushnell, MC; Farrar, JT; Galer, BS; Haythornthwaite, JA; Hewitt, DJ; Loeser, JD; Max, MB; Saltarelli, M; Schmader, KE; Stein, C; Thompson, D; Turk, DC; Wallace, MS; Watkins, LR; Weinstein, SM. Advances in neuropathic pain. *Arch Neurol* 2003, 60, 1524-1534.

Elliott, AM; Smith, BH; Penny, KI; Smith, WC; Chambers WA. The epidemiology of chronic pain in the community. *Lancet* 1999, 354, 1248-1252.

Eriksen, J; Jensen, MK; Sjøgren, P; Ekholm, O; Rasmussen NK. Epidemiology of chronic non-malignant pain in Denmark. *Pain* 2003, 106, 221-228

Fatt, P; Katz, B. Spontaneous activity at motor nerve endings. *J Physiol* (Lond) 1952, 117, 109-128.

FDA Consum. New drug for neuropathic pain. *FDA Consum* 2004, 38, 2.

Fertuck, HC; Salpeter, MM. Localization of acetylcholine receptor by 125I-labeled alpha-bungarotoxin binding at mouse motor endplates. *Proc Natl Acad Sci* 1974, 71, 1376-1378.

Flores, CM; Rogers, SW; Pabreza, LA; Wolfe, BB; Kellar, KJ. A subtype of nicotinic cholinergic receptor in rat brain is composed of alpha 4 and beta 2 subunits and is up-regulated by chronic nicotine treatment. *Mol Pharmacol* 1992, 41, 31-37.

Flores, CM; DeCamp, RM; Kilo, S; Rogers, SW; Hargreaves, KM. Neuronal nicotinic receptor expression in sensory neurons of the rat trigeminal ganglion: demonstration of αlpha3beta4, a novel subtype in the mammalian nervous system. *J Neurosci* 1996, 16, 7892-7901.

Gauvin, DM; Decker, MW; Meyer, MD; Sullivan, JP; Honore, P. Effects of ABT-594, a neuronal nicotinic receptor agonist, in a rodent model of post-operative pain. *Soc Neurosci Abstr* 2003, 2003, 384.5.

Gilbert ,SD; Clark, TM; Flores, CM. Antihyperalgesic activity of epibatidine in the formalin model of facial pain. *Pain* 2001, 89, 159-165.

Gotti C, Clementi F. Neuronal nicotinic receptors: from structure to pathology. *Prog Neurobiol* 2004, 74, 363-396.

Hagan, RM; Domeney, AM; Martin, BR; Damaj, MI; Kellar, KJ; Dukat, M; Simsek, R; Glennon, RA. BTG-102, a novel nicotinic analgesic agent. *Soc Neurosci Abstr* 2003, 2003, 693.11.

Hansson, PT; Dickenson, AH. Pharmacological treatment of peripheral neuropathic pain conditions based on shared commonalities despite multiple etiologies. *Pain* 2005, 113, 251-254.

Harden, N; Cohen M. Unmet needs in the management of neuropathic pain. *J Pain Symptom Manage* 2003, 25, S12-S17.

Hochberg, MC. Treatment of rheumatoid arthritis and osteoarthritis with Cox-2-selective inhibitors: a managed care perspective. *Amer J Manag Care* 2002, 8, S502-S517.

Iwamoto, ET. Antinociception after nicotine administration into the mesopontine tegmentum of rats: evidence for muscarinic actions. *J Pharmacol Exp Ther* 1989, 251, 412-421.

Iwamoto, ET. Characterization of the antinociception induced by nicotine in the pedunculopontine tegmental nucleus and the nucleus raphe magnus. *J Pharmacol Exp Ther* 1991, 257, 120-133.

Jacobson, L; Mariano, A. General considerations of chronic pain. In: Loeser JD, Butler SH, Chapman CR, editors. *Bonica's Management of Pain. 3rd edition*. Baltimore, MD: Lippincott Williams & Wilkins; 2001;241-254.

Jamner, LD; Girdler, SS; Shapiro, D; Jarvik, ME. Pain inhibition, nicotine, and gender. *Exp Clin Psychopharmacol* 1998, 6, 96-106.

Jordan, KG; Letchworth, SR; Traina, VM; Gatto, GJ; Bencherif, M. TC-2696: an orally, effective neuronal nicotinic receptor modulator with antinociceptive and antihyperalgesic/antiallodynic activity. *Soc Neurosci Abstr* 2004, 63.11.

Kesingland, AC; Gentry, CT; Panesar, MS; Bowes, MA; Vernier, JM; Cube, R; Walker, K; Urban, L. Analgesic prodile of the nicotine actetylcholine receptor agonists, (+)-epibatidine and ABT-594 in models of persistent inflammatory and neuropathic pain. *Pain* 2000, 86, 113-118.

Khan, IM; Buerkle, H; Taylor, P; Yaksh, TL. Nociceptive and antinociceptive responses to intrathecally administered nicotinic agonists. *Neuropharmacology* 1998, 37, 1515-1525.

Khan, IM; Osaka, H; Stanislaus, S; Calvo, RM; Deerinck, T; Yaksh, TL; Taylor, P. Nicotinic acetylcholine receptor distribution in relation to spinal neurotransmission pathways. *J Comp Neurol* 2003, 467, 44-59.

Leikola-Pelho, T; Jackson, DM. Preferential stimulation of locomotor activity by ventral tegmental microinjections of (-)-nicotine. *Pharmacol Toxicol* 1992, 70, 50-52.

Lynch, JJ 3rd; Wade, CL; Mikusa, JP; Decker, MW; Honore, P. ABT-594 (a nicotinic acetylcholine agonist): anti-allodynia in a rat chemotherapy-induced pain model. *Eur J Pharmacol* 2005, 509, 43-48.

Marubio, LM; del Mar Arroyo-Jimenez, M; Cordero-Erausquin, M; Léna, C; Le Novère, N; de Kerchove d-Exaerde, A; Huchet, M; Damaj, MI; Changeux, J-P. Reduced antinociception in mice lacking neuronal nicotinic receptor subunits. *Nature* 1999, 398, 805-810.

McCaffery, M; Portenoy, RK. Overview of three groups of analgesics. In: McCaffery M, Pasero C, editors. *Pain Clinical Manual. 2nd edition*. St. Louis, MO: Mosby Inc; 1999a; 103-128.

McCaffery, M; Portenoy, RK. Nonopioids: acetaminophen and nonsteroidal antiinflammatory drugs (NSAIDs). In: McCaffery M, Pasero C, editors. *Pain Clinical Manual. 2nd edition*. St. Louis, MO: Mosby Inc; 1999b; 129-160.

McCleane G. Pharmacological management of neuropathic pain. *CNS Drugs* 2003, 17, 1031-1043.

McCleane G. Pharmacological strategies in relieving neuropathic pain. *Exp Opin Pharmacother* 2004 5, 1299-1312.

McMahon, SB; Wall, PD. Receptive fields of rat lamina 1 projection cells move to incorporate a nearby region of injury. *Pain* 1984, 19, 235-247.

Merskey, H; Bugduk, N. Classification of Chronic Pain. *Descriptions of Chronic Pain Syndromes and Definitions of Pain Terms. 2nd ed.* Seattle, WA: IASP Press, 1994.

Meyer, RA; Campbell, JN; Raja, SN. Peripheral neural mechanisms of cutaneous hyperalgesia. In: Fields HL, Dubner R, Cervero F. *Advances in Pain Research and Therapy. Vol. 9*. New York: Raven; 1985; 53-71.

Millan, MJ. The induction of pain: an integrative review. Prog Neurobiol 1999, 57, 1-164.

Pappagallo, M. Newer antiepileptic drugs: possible uses in the treatment of neuropathic pain and migraine. *Clin Ther* 2003, 25, 2506-2538.

Pasero, C; Portenoy, RK; McCaffery, M. Opioid analgesics. In: McCaffery M, Pasero C, editors. *Pain Clinical Manual. 2nd edition*. St. Louis, MO: Mosby Inc; 1999; 161-299.

Picciotto, MR; Zoli, M; Rimondini, R; Lena, C; Marubio, LM; Pich, EM; Fuxe, K; Changeux, JP. Acetylcholine receptors containing the beta2 subunit are involved in the reinforcing properties of nicotine. *Nature* 1998, 391, 173-177.

Pickworth, WB; Bunker, EB; Henningfield, JE. Transdermal nicotine: reduction of smoking with minimal abuse liability. *Psychopharmacology* 1994, 115, 9-14.

Plenge, P; Mellerup, ET; Wortwein, G. Characterization of epibatidine binding to medial habenula: potential role in analgesia. *J Pharmacol Exp Ther* 2002, 302, 759-765.

Portenoy, RK; Lesage, P. Management of cancer pain. *Lancet* 1999, 353, 1695-1700.

Portenoy, RK. Current pharmacotherapy of chronic pain. *J Pain Symptom Manage* 2000, 19, S16-S20.

Radek, RJ; Curzon, P; Decker, MW. Supraspinal and systemic administration of the nicotinic-cholinergic agonist (±)-epibatidine has inhibitory effects on C-fiber reflexes in the rat. *Brain Res Bull* 2004, 64, 323-330.

Rao, TS; Sacaan, AI; Menzaghi, FM; Reid, RT; Adams, PB; Correa, LD; Whelan, KT; Vernier, JM. Pharmacological characterization of SIB-1663, a conformationally rigid analog of nicotine. *Brain Res* 2004, 1003, 42-53.

Rashid, MH; Ueda H. Neuropathy-specific analgesic action of intrathecal nicotinic agonists and its spinal GABA-mediated mechanism. *Brain Res* 2002, 953, 53-62.

Rau, H; Schweizer, R; Zhuang, P; Pauli, P; Brody, S; Larbig, W; Heinle, H; Muller, M; Elbert, T; Dworkin, B. Cigarette smoking, blood lipids, and baroreceptor-modulated nociception. *Psychopharmacology* 1993, 110, 337-341.

Rueter, LE; Kohlhaas, KL; Curzon, P; Surowy, CS; Meyer, MD. Peripheral and central sites of action for A-85380 in the spinal nerve ligation model of neuropathic pain. *Pain* 2003, 103, 269-276.

Rueter, LE; Meyer, MD; Decker, MW. Spinal mechanisms underlying A-85380-induced effects on acute thermal pain. *Brain Res* 2000, 872, 93-101.

Seguela, P; Wadiche, J; Dineley-Miller, K; Dani, JA; Patrick, JW. Molecular cloning, functional properties, and distribution of rat brain alpha 7: a nicotinic cation channel highly permeable to calcium. *J Neurosci* 1993, 13, 596-604.

Slade, J; Henningfield, JE. Tobacco product regulation: context and issues. *Food Drug Law J* 1998, 53, 43-74.

Smith, PA. Neuropathic pain: drug targets for current and future interventions. *Drug News Perspect* 2004, 17, 5-17.

Sullivan, JP; Bannon, AW. Epibatidine: pharmacological properties of a novel nicotinic acetycholine receptor agonist and analgesic agent. *CNS Drug Rev* 1996, 2, 21-39.

Treede, RD; Meyer, RA; Raja, SN; Campbell, JN. Peripheral and central mechanisms of cutaneous hyperalgesia. *Prog Neurobiol* 1992,38, 397-421.

Tsuda, M; Inoue, K; Salter, MW. Neuropathic pain and spinal microglia: a big problem from molecules in "small" glia. *Trends Neurosci* 2005, 28, 101-107.

Turk, DC; Okifuji, A. Pain Terms and taxonomies of pain. In: Loeser JD, Butler SH, Chapman CR, editorss. *Bonica's Management of Pain. 3rd edition*. Baltimore, MD: Lippincott Williams & Wilkins; 2001; 17-25.

Vincler, MA; Eisenach, JC. Knock down of the αalpha5 nicotinic acetylcholine receptor in spinal nerve-ligated rats alleviates mechanial allodynia. *Pharmacol Biochem Behav* 2005, 80, 135-143.

Wang, N; Orr-Urtreger, A; Korczyn, AD. The role of neuronal nicotinic acetylcholine receptor subunits in autonomic ganglia: lessons from knockout mice. *Prog Neurobiol* 2002, 68, 341-360.

Watkins, LR; Milligan, ED; Maier, SF. Spinal cord glia: new players in pain. *Pain* 2001, 93, 201-205.

Whiteaker, P; Peterson, CG; Xu, W; McIntosh, JM; Paylor, R; Beaudet, AL; Collins, AC; Marks, MJ. Involvement of the alpha3 subunit in central nicotinic binding populations. *J Neurosci* 2002, 22, 2522-2529.

Woolf, CJ. Evidence for a central component of post-injury pain hypersensitivity. *Nature* 1983, 306, 686–688.

Woolf, CJ; Thompson, SW. The induction and maintenance of central sensitization is dependent on N-methyl-D-aspartic acid receptor activation: implications for the treatment of post-injury pain hypersensitivity states. *Pain* 1991, 44, 293–299.

Woolf, CJ; Salter, MW. Neuronal plasticity: increasing the gain in pain. *Science* 2000, 288, 1765-1769.

Xiao, H-S; Huang, Q-H; Zhang, F-X; Bao, L; Lu, Y-J; Guo, C; Yang, L; Huang, W-J; Fu, G; Xu, S-H; Cheng, X-P; Yan, Q; Zhu, Z-D; Zhang, X; Chen, Z; Han, Z-G; Zhang, X. Identification of gene expression profile of dorsal root ganglion in the rat peripheral axotomy model of neuropathic pain. *Proc Natl Acad Sci* 2002, 99, 8360-8365.

Yang, L; Zhang, F-X; Huang, F; Lu, Y-J; Li, G-D; Bao, L; Xiao, H-S; Zhang, X. Peripheral nerve injury induces trans-synaptic modification of channels, receptors and signal pathways in rat dorsal spinal cord. *Eur J Neurosci* 2004, 19, 871-883.

Zarrindast, MR; Baghdadi, B; Sahebgharani, M. Potentiation of imipramine-induced antinociception by nicotine in the formalin test. *Eur Neuropscyhopharmacol* 2004, 14, 71-76.

In Frontiers in Pain Research
Editor: Alexandre Lucas, pp.101-111

ISBN 1-59454-828-5

Chapter 5

SPINAL CORD STIMULATION: MECHANISMS AND CLINICAL APPLICATION

Milan P. Stojanovic
Interventional Pain Program, Massachusetts General Hospital,
Harvard Medical School, Boston, Massachusetts

ABSTRACT

In 1965 Melzak and Wall gate control theory proposed that stimulation of A-beta fibers modulates the dorsal horn "gate" and therefore reduces the nociceptive input from periphery. The gate control theory sparked clinician's interest and already by 1967 Shealy and colleagues published the first report on spinal cord stimulation (SCS) in humans. The first SCS was placed intrathecaly via open laminotomy. Although effective in many patients, the underdeveloped hardware significantly slowed down the progress of SCS in the 1970's. With significant improvement in hardware design and simplifaction of trial techniques with introducing epidural approach in 1980's, the SCS gained in popularity and now is routinely used in clinical practice to treat many chronic pain conditions.

Over the last two decades, many clinical outcome studies have supported the use of SCS for chronic pain. The SCS is particularly beneficial in reducing pain in patients with lumbar and cervical radiculopathy and complex regional pain syndrome (CRPS). Several randomized studies have shown the clear advantages of SCS over re-operation in patients who failed back surgery. Recently, there is good evidence that SCS may be very beneficial for treatment of chest pain due to coronary artery disease in patients who fail conservative treatment options.

Over the last two decades, the understanding of SCS mechanisms of action evolved significantly. Rather than explained by gate control theory, it seems that mechanisms of SCS action are more complex. These mechanisms may involve increased dorsal horn inhibitory action of GABA, adenosine and the disinhibition of descending analgesia pathways originating in periaqueductal gray (PAG). Due to these modulatory actions in the CNS, the SCS is often named "Neuromodulation."

The history of SCS development is a perfect example of how new ideas can spark expansion of useful clinical application.

INTRODUCTION

The neurodestructive procedures used to treat pain were mostly abandoned due to our better understanding of neurobiology of pain. Initial pain relief obtained by surgical section of certain pain pathways in the central nervous system (CNS) or peripheral nerves is usually followed by a much longer period of increased pain due to permanent changes in the nervous system induced by nerve injury. For these reasons, many of neurodestructive procedures are now replaced by spinal cord stimulation (SCS) which is minimally invasive and reversible.

The first time in history the electrical power (torpedo fish) was used for medical treatment was in 600 BC. The first report of electrical stimulation of the human brain was reported in 1874. The first implantation of brain electrodes took place in 1948 for treatment of psychiatric disorders.

However, the use of electrical power for pain relief has not emerged until 1950's. Early trials have been unsuccessful until Melzack and Wall proposed the gate theory of pain in 1965 [1]. Based on this theory, Shealy and associates published the first report of the SCS in 1967 [2]. These initial SCS implants in humans involved open intrathecal implantation of electrodes via laminotomy. However, the lack of adequate hardware and paucity of clinical outcome studies have significantly slowed down the development of neurostimulation in the 1970's.

Over the last two decades, the hardware technology and implantation techniques significantly improved. Each implantation of the SCS system is preceded by several days of outpatient SCS trial. During the trial period, the patients are able to test the SCS in their daily surroundings. Only if they are fully satisfied with the trial, the permanent stimulator implant is planned.

Many recent clinical studies fully support the SCS for various forms of chronic pain. This applies in particular for treatment of lumbar radiculopathy, failed back surgery syndrome and complex regional pain syndrome (CRPS).

When deciding on any invasive treatment for chronic pain, the risk/benefit ratio is the single most important factor to consider before a decision is made to perform the procedure. With improvements of hardware technology, the risk/benefit ratio of SCS become very low. Because of these high safety margins one should consider trying the SCS before many other treatment options, such as opioid medications, are considered.

Over the last decade, the new indications for the SCS emerged. Recent clinical studies support the SCS for treatment of chest pain due to coronary artery disease and pain induced by peripheral vascular disease. The patients with occipital neuralgia and pelvic pain may also benefit from peripheral implantation of stimulating electrodes.

MECHANISMS OF SCS PAIN NEUROMODULATION

Melzak and Wall gate control theory was a basic principle upon which the first experiments of SCS were performed [1]. Their initial theory proposed that stimulation of A-beta fibers modulates the dorsal horn "gate" and, therefore, reduces the nociceptive input from periphery. Later, several studies demonstrated that dorsal horn neuronal activity caused by peripheral noxious stimuli could be inhibited by concomitant stimulation of the dorsal columns [3]. However, recent studies revealed that alternate mechanisms may be also responsible for SCS action [4,5,6].

Several animal studies support the suppressive effect of SCS on tactile allodynia [7]. The tactile allodynia is mediated via Aβ fibers and represents the state of central hyperexcitability [8]. Allodynic animals seem to have lower extracellular levels of GABA [9]. One of the proposed mechanisms of SCS action involves increased dorsal horn inhibitory action of GABA [10]. The allodynia suppressive effect of SCS was abolished by GABA antagonists in rats [11]. On the other hand, intrathecal administration of $GABA_B$ agonist, baclofen, enhances the antinociceptive action of SCS in an animal model [12].

Several other putative mechanisms may be responsible for pain relief induced by SCS. Recent animal and human studies revealed a potential role of adenosine in SCS mechanisms of action. Intrathecal administration of $adenosine_A$ receptor agonist was found to have a potentiating effect with SCS and also a synergistic effect with baclofen [4]. The disinhibition of descending analgesia pathways originating in periaqueductal gray (PAG) can be another explanation of SCS action [13] and so is SCS induced release of serotonin and substance P [14]. In rats in which SCS failed to suppress tactile hypersensitivity, the combination of SCS and a subeffective dose of clonidine appeared to be highly synergistic, and it markedly attenuated the hypersensitivity. These results suggest that small doses of IT clonidine may be combined with SCS in neuropathic pain patients who do not obtain satisfactory relief with SCS alone [15].

In patients with peripheral vascular disease, SCS may abolish peripheral ischemic pain by rebalancing the oxygen need and supply and preventing ischemia and by suppressing the sympathetic activity via α-adrenorecptors [4,5,6]. At increased amplitudes of SCS the nitric oxide dependent release of calcitonin gene-related peptide (CGRP) may be more responsible for vasodilatation effect [16]. Better survival of skin flaps during SCS seems to be due to the CGRP mediated mechanism [17]. However, no changes in peripheral blood flow were documented despite excellent pain relief with the SCS (18).

Angina due to coronary artery disease (CAD) and end-stage myocardial ischemia are excellent indications for the SCS. A likely mechanism for pain relief in CAD is redistribution of the coronary blood flow from regions with normal perfusion in favor of regions with impaired myocardial perfusion [19]. Other possible mechanism of SCS action in CAD is suppression of excitatory effects of myocardial ischemia on intrinsic cardiac neurons [20]. The SCS may reduce the incidence of ventricular arrhythmias in post infarction animal model [21].

Functional magnetic resonance imaging (fMRI) studies have revealed patterns of alterations in pain processing in human brains induced by SCS. This includes increased activity in human somatosensory cortex (SI and SII areas) contralateral to the side of pain and cingulate gyri with SCS activation. The somatosensory cortex activation is amplitude dependent (22). These brain areas activated by SCS correspond to CNS pain pathways involved in processing of somatosensory (SI, SII) and affective components (cingulate gyri) of pain.

Clinical Indications for SCS Tratment

One of the main advantages of SCS is its non-neurodestructive nature. As opposed to neuroablation and many other neurosurgical procedures, the SCS is a reversible, minimally invasive procedure. Recently, many studies have confirmed good clinical outcomes of SCS and helped its increased popularity.

Lumbar Radiculopathy

The most common indication for SCS placement in United States today is lumbar radiculopathy, commonly associated with Failed Back Surgery Syndrome (FBSS)

The outcomes of SCS for this indication improved over the last two decades while complication rates declined [23]. The FBSS is an often a type of radicular pain defined as persistent pain after attempted surgical treatment for low back pain. In patients who failed medical management, physical therapy and nerve blocks, the SCS may be the best treatment choice. Many studies are supporting the role of SCS in these patients, emphasizing its advantages over re-operation [24,25]. Some cases of lumbar radiculopathy may respond better to SCS lead placement directly through neural foramina (retrograde lead placement) [26]. Reported success rates in treating FBSS vary from 12% to 88%. A systematic review of literature related to SCS and FBSS by Turner *et al.* [27] revealed that an average of 59% patients had ≥50% pain relief with SCS.

Isolated, "Axial" Low Back Pain

The use of SCS for axial low back pain (without radicular component) has been controversial. Recent studies seem to provide better support revealing over 50% success rates [28]. The single electrodes seem to have clear advantages over the dual electrodes for treatment of axial pain [28].

Complex Regional Pain Syndrome (CRPS)

Dr. Mitchell was the first to describe a CRPS in 1864, better known by its previous terms reflex sympathetic dystrophy (RSD) or causalgia [29]. The CRPS I and II responds well to SCS with reported effectiveness range from 50-91% [30,31]. The best candidates for SCS are patients with upper or lower extremity pain. In a randomized trial by Kemler *et al.*, patients with CRPS who received SCS treatment and physical therapy had better improvement (56% success rate) than patients who received physical therapy alone with the confirmed results in a two-year follow-up of the same study [31,32].

The subgroup of CRPS, a sympathetically maintained pain, seems to respond better to SCS than sympathetically independent pain. Recent study by Hord et al. reported that patients with good response to sympathetic block before SCS are more likely to have a positive response during their SCS trial and long-term pain relief after placement of permanent SCS device [33].

Diabetic Neuropathy

In certain cases of diabetic neuropathy the SCS can provide pain relief and help to salvage the affected limb. Due to a higher infection risk, special precaution in patients with diabetic neuropathy should be used when SCS implantation is anticipated [34]. The patients with an increase in transcutaneous oxygen tension (TcpO(2)) during SCS trial seem to respond better to SCS [35].

Post Herpetic Neuralgia

The scientific evidence on efficacy of SCS for postherpetic neuralgia (PHN) is scarce. However, the recent study showed excellent outcomes with this modality [36]. In the United States, the SCS treatment of PHN is considered investigational. Further randomized studies are needed to better establish a role of SCS in this form of neuropathic pain.

Other Neuropathic Pain States

The SCS have shown good outcomes in many cases of neuropathic pain as mentioned previously (CRPS, diabetic neuropathy, PHN). However, many cases of deafferentation pain including phantom limb syndrome and cases of spinal cord injury do not seem to respond well to the SCS, most likely due to a cortical re-organization of pain processing.

Coronary Artery Disease

Cases of anginal pain may respond well to SCS [37]. The best indication for SCS trial is angina refractory to pharmacologic and surgical treatments. An increase in exercise capacity, reduction in anginal complaints, decreased use of short-acting nitrates and improved quality of life has been demonstrated in patients with ischemic heart disease treated with SCS. In 60% of the patients, SCS was effective five years after implantation, and more than 80% patients benefited from SCS for at least one year [38].

In certain patients with severe angina pectoris, the SCS proved advantageous to the coronary artery bypass surgery as shown in randomized trial setting in certain patients with severe angina pectoris [39].

The fear of potential increase in myocardial damage does not seem to be justified since the SCS does not completely abolish anginal pain. It only raises the anginal threshold and does not seem to have negative effect on left ventricular ejection fraction nor cardiac arrhythmias [40]. As already mentioned, the SCS has been shown to reduce the incidence of ventricular arrhythmias in a post infarction animal model [21].

Peripheral Vascular Disease

Several studies reported excellent pain relief in patients with peripheral vascular disease with SCS ranging from 60-100%. Besides providing pain relief, SCS may increase the peripheral blood flow, promote ulcer healing and potentially contribute to limb salvage. Studies have shown that an increase in TcpO2 during the first two weeks of post implantation predicts future limb salvage, and ischemic ulcers of less than 3cm^2 are likely to heal with SCS treatment [41,42,43].

Contraindications

Before SCS implantation, a psychological evaluation of the patient is recommended since implantation of the SCS in severe psychiatric disease is contraindicated and certain psychological tests have been shown to correlate with outcomes to SCS [44]. One should use caution in SCS placement in patients with cervical and thoracic spinal canal stenosis. This applies in particular to dual lead and neurosurgically implanted systems. Infection, drug abuse and some coagulopathies may be the contraindications for SCS placement.

The overall cost of SCS can actually be lower than conservative management options. The costs of medications, emergency room visits, multiple physician visits, x-rays, absence from work can easily surpass the cost of SCS implant. Bell and colleagues have shown that for those patients for whom SCS is clinically efficacious, the SCS pays for itself within 2.1 years [45].

IMPLANTATION LOGISTICS AND HARDWARE

The SCS hardware consists of leads, extension and implantable pulse generator (IPG). The leads are placed in the epidural space usually in thoracic and cervical spine for leg and arm pain coverage, respectively. The actual stimulation occurs from electrodes, placed at the distal end of the lead. An electrical field from SCS leads/electrodes reaches the dorsal columns of the spinal cord and modulates its pain transmission.

The SCS leads are placed at the desired spinal level in the epidural space. The most common placement is done percutaneously under fluoroscopic guidance . It has been shown that the spinal cord midline and vertebral midline are apart by at least 1-2mm in 40% of the patients. Bartolat and colleagues found that only 27% of paresthesia was felt symmetrically when the stimulating contacts were perfectly located at the radiological midline [46].

The anatomical position of SCS lead can influence the pain relief and SCS "coverage." For chronic low back pain treatment the SCS electrode leads are placed in the thoracic epidural space, with a lead tip location at T8-T10 level, and for arm pain, the SCS lead tip is placed at C2-3 level. The CSF thickness is the main factor in determining the perception threshold and paresthesia coverage in spinal cord stimulation: an increasing thickness raises the threshold and reduces the coverage.

SCS Trial

One of the major advantages of SCS is the safety and simplicity of the SCS trial. The percutaneous SCS trial is a minimally invasive procedure and can positively predict a long-term outcome in 50-70% of cases. The trial allows the patients to evaluate the SCS analgesic activity in their everyday surroundings for several days before deciding to have permanent SCS implant.

Permanent SCS Implant

While the trial is usually done in the outpatient clinic setting, the permanent SCS placement is reserved for the operating room. Under local anesthesia and IV sedation, the skin incision is made along the lumbar insertion site where stimulator lead is placed and anchored to the skin. At separate subcutanous pocket is made for a pulse generator in the gluteal or abdominal area. The SCS lead is then connected with the IPG through an extension cable tunneled through the skin.

The permanent SCS implant can be achieved by placing the percutaneous lead via epidural needle or "paddle" lead via open laminotomy. The paddle electrodes are larger, can be anchored directly to the dura, potentially minimizing migration and providing better stimulation coverage in some cases [47].

There are three types of IPG's: a) the completely implanted IPG containing a battery; b) the IPG supplied by external power through the radio frequency antenna applied to the skin; c) the completely implanted IPG containing an externally rechargeable battery.

For the completely implanted IPG, the batteries have to be changed every 3-6 years. The battery life depends on the total time the stimulator is used and the stimulation amplitude. The externally powered and rechargeable IPG's have the advantage over the implanted ones in patients requiring higher amplitudes of stimulation, which would otherwise deplete the implanted batteries in a short period of time.

Complications

Serious SCS complications are very rare. The most common surgical complication is hardware failure (migration, lead and IPG failure) and infection. Antibiotic prohylaxis is warranted before the SCS implantation.

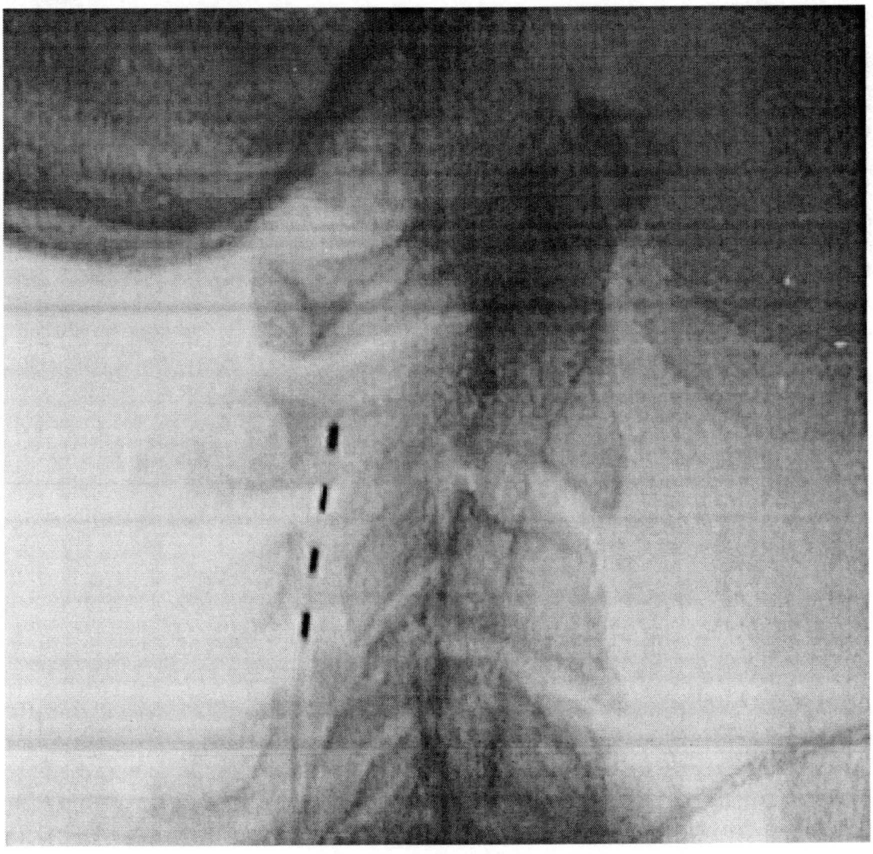

Figure 1.

CONLUSION

The SCS is an excellent treatment choice, particularly in patients with lumbar radiculopathy, CRPS, and some patients with CAD and peripheral vascular disease. The main advantages of the SCS over the other treatment options are its favorable risk/benefit ratio which are supported in clinical studies and the reversibility of this treatment. More studies are needed to better define patient selection criteria and outcome predictors to this treatment modality.

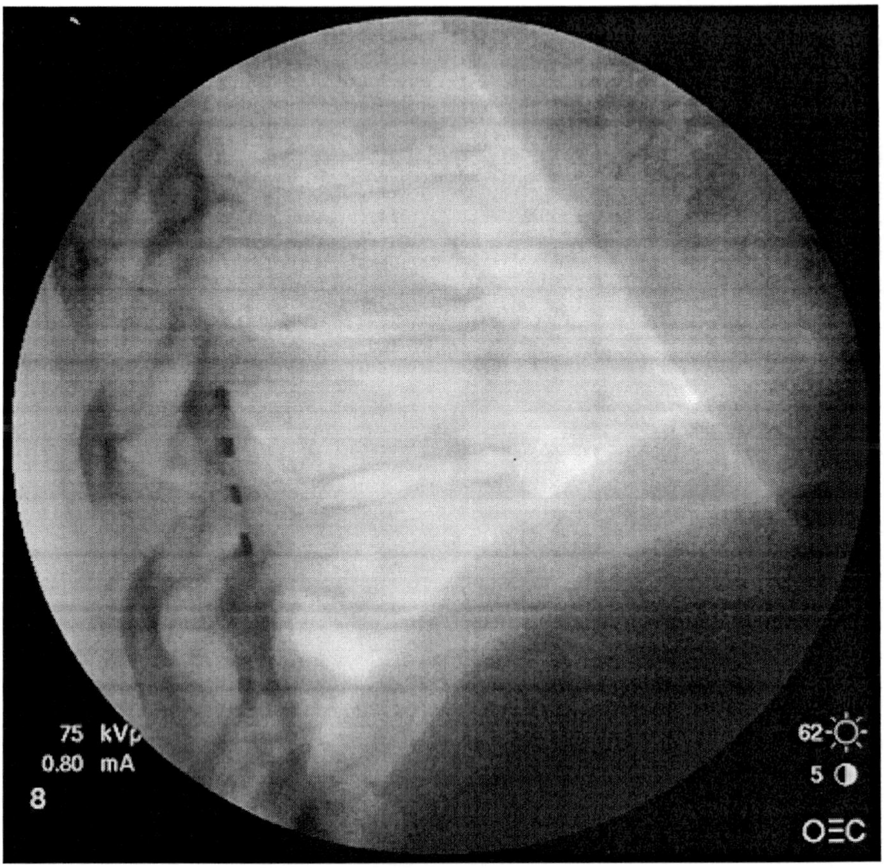

Figure 2.

REFERENCES

[1] Melzack R, Wall P. Pain Mechanism: a new theory. *Science* 1965, 150:951-979.

[2] Shealy C, Mortimer J, Reswick J. Electrical inhibition of pain by stimulation of the dorsal columns: preliminary report. *Anesth Analg* 1967, 46:489-491.

[3] Dubuisson D. Effect of dorsal-column stimulation on gelatinosa and marginal neurons of cat spinal cord. *J Neurosurg.* 1989; 70. 257-265.

[4] Meyerson B, Linderoth B. Mechanisms of spinal cord stimulation in neuropathic pain. *Neurolog Res.* 2000, 22: 285-292.

[5] Linderoth B, Foreman R. Physiology of Spinal Cord Stimulation: Review and Update. *Neuromodulation* 1999, (2- 3): 150-164.

[6] Stiller C-O, Linderoth B, O'Connor W et al. Repeated spinal cord stimulation decreases the extracellular level of gamma-aminobutiric acid in periaqueductal grey matter of freely moving rats. *Brain Res* 1995; 699: 231-241.

[7] Yakhnitsa V, Linderoth B, Meyerson BA. Spinal cord stimulation attenuates dorsal horn neuronal hyperexcitability in a rat model of mononeuropathy. *Pain.*1999, 79(2-3):223-33.

[8] Bennett G. An animal model of neuropathic pain: A review. *Muscle Nerve* 1993; 16: 1040-1048.

[9] Stiller C-O, Cui C-G, O'Connor WT et al. Release of GABA in the dorsal horn and suppression of tactile allodynia by spinal cord stimulation in mononeuropathic rats. *Neurosurg*1996; 39: 367-375.

[10] Cui JG, O'Connor WT, Ungerstedt U et al. Spinal cord stimulation attenuates dorsal horn release of excitatory amino acids in mononeuropathy via a GABAergic mechanism. *Pain;* 1997:73:87-95.

[11] Cui JG, Linderoth B, Meyerson BA. Effects of spinal cord stimulation on touch evoked allodynia involve GABAergic mechanisms. An experimental study in mononeuropathic rat. *Pain* 1996;66:287-295.

[12] Meyerson BA, Cui J-G, Yakhnitsa V et al. Modulation of spinal pain mechanisms by spinal cord stimulation and the potential role of adjuvant pharmacotherapy. *Stereotact Funct Neurosurg* 1997; 68: 129-140.

[13] Stiller C-O, Linderoth B, O'Connor W et al. Repeated spinal cord stimulation decreases the extracellular level of gamma-aminobutiric acid in periaqueductal grey matter of freely moving rats. *Brain Res* 1995; 699: 231-241.

[14] Linderoth B, Gazelius B, Franck J et al. Dorsal column stimulation induces release of serotonin and substance P in the cat dorsal horn. *Neurosurg* 1992, 31:289-296.

[15] Schechtman G, Meyerson BA, Linderoth B. Intrathecal clonidine potentiates suppression of tactile hypersensitivity by spinal cord stimulation in a model of neuropathy. *Anesthesia & Analgesia.* 2004;99(1):135-9.

[16] Croom JE, Foreman RD, Chandler MJ et al. Cutaneous vasodilatation during dorsal column stimulation is mediated by dorsal roots and CGRP. *Am J Physiol* 1997; 272:H950-H957.

[17] Gheradini G, Lundenberg T, Cui J-G et al. Spinal cord stimulation improves survival in ischemic skin flaps: an experimental study of the possible mediation by calcitonin gene-related peptide. *Plast Reconstr Surg.* 103(4):1221-8, 1999.

[18] Kemler MA. Barendse GA. van Kleef M. et al. Pain relief in complex regional pain syndrome due to spinal cord stimulation does not depend on vasodilation. *Anesthesiology.* 2000;92(6):1653-60.

[19] Hautvast RWM, Dejongste MJL, Blansma PK, et al. Spinal cord stimulation causes redistribution in myocardial perfusion during dypiridamole stress testing in patients with refractory angina pectoris as assessed by 13 NH3-positron emission tomography. *Am J Cardiol* 1996, 77:462-467.

[20] Foreman RD. Linderoth B. Ardell JL et al. Modulation of intrinsic cardiac neurons by spinal cord stimulation: implications for its therapeutic use in angina pectoris. *Cardiovascular Research*.2000, 47(2):367-75.

[21] Issa ZF, Zhou X, Ujehlyi et al. Thoracic spinal cord stimulation reduces the risk of ischemic ventricular arrhythmias in a postinfarction heart failure canine model. *Circulation*.2005;111(24):3217-20.

[22] Kiriakopoulos ET. Tasker RR. Nicosia S. et al. Functional magnetic resonance imaging: a potential tool for the evaluation of spinal cord stimulation: technical case report *Neurosurg*. 1997;41(2):501-4.

[23] North RB. Wetzel FT. Spinal cord stimulation for chronic pain of spinal origin: a valuable long-term solution. *Spine*. 2002;15;27(22):2584-91; discussion 2592.

[24] North RB, Ewend MG, Lawton MT. Failed back surgery syndrome: Five year follow up after spinal cord stimulator implantation. A prospective, randomized study design. *Neurosurg* 1991;28:692-699.

[25] North RB. Kidd DH. Farrokhi F. Piantadosi SA. Spinal cord stimulation versus repeated lumbosacral spine surgery for chronic pain: a randomized, controlled trial. *Neurosurgery*.2005; 56(1):98-106; discussion 106-6.

[26] Alo KM, Yland MJ, Redko V et al. Lumbar and sacral nerve root stimulation (NRS) in the treatment of chronic pain, a novel anathomic approach and neuro stimulation technique. *Neuromodulation* 1999;2:19-27.

[27] Turner JA, Loeser JD, Bell KG. Spinal cord stimulation for chronic low back pain: A systematic literature synthesis. *Neurosurg* 1995; 37:1088-1096.

[28] North RB. Kidd DH. Olin J. Sieracki JM. Farrokhi F. Petrucci L. Cutchis PN. Spinal cord stimulation for axial low back pain: a prospective, controlled trial comparing dual with single percutaneous electrodes. *Spine*. 2005; 30(12):1412-8.

[29] Mitchell SW, Morehouse G, Keen WW. Gunshot wounds and other injuries to the nerves. Philadelphia: *J.B. Lippincott*, 1864.

[30] Kumar K, Toth C, Nath RK. Spinal cord stimulation is effective in reflex sympathetic dystrophy. *Neurosurgery* 1997. 40:503-509.

[31] Kemler MA, Barendse GAM, van Kleef M et al. Spinal Cord Stimulation in Patients with Chronic Reflex Sympathetic Dystrophy. *N Engl J Med*, 2000, 343:618-624.

[32] Kemler MA, De Vet HC, Barendse GA, Van Den Wildenberg FA, Van Kleef M. The effect of spinal cord stimulation in patients with chronic reflex sympathetic dystrophy: two years' follow-up of the randomized controlled trial. *Ann Neurol*. 2004;55(1):13-8.

[33] Hord ED, Cohen SP, Cosgrove GR, Ahmed SU, Vallejo R, Chang Y, Stojanovic MP. The predictive value of sympathetic block for the success of spinal cord stimulation. *Neurosurgery*. 2003 Sep;53(3):626-32; discussion 632-3.

[34] Torrens JK. Stanley PJ. Ragunathan PL.et al. Risk of infection with electrical spinal-cord stimulation [letter; comment]. *Lancet* 1997,349(9053):729.

[35] Petrakis IE. Sciacca V. Spinal cord stimulation in diabetic lower limb critical ischaemia: transcutaneous oxygen measurement as predictor for treatment success. *Eur J Vasc Endovasc Surg*. 2000 19(6):587-92.

[36] Harke, H. et al. Spinal Cord Stimulation in Postherpetic Neuralgia and in Acute Herpes Zoster *Pain*. 2002; 94(3); 694-700.

[37] DeJongste MJ. Spinal cord stimulation for ischemic heart disease. *Neurol Res* 2000; 22(3):293-.298.

[38] Hautvast RW. DeJongste MJ. Staal MJ et al. Spinal cord stimulation in chronic intractable angina pectoris: a randomized, controlled efficacy study. *Am Heart J* 1998, 136(6):1114-20.

[39] Mannheimer C. Eliasson T. Augustinsson LE. Et al. Electrical stimulation versus coronary artery bypass surgery in severe angina pectoris: the ESBY study. *Circulation.*1998, 97(12):1157-63.

[40] Jessurun GA. Ten Vaarwerk IA. DeJongste MJ et al Sequelae of spinal cord stimulation for refractory angina pectoris. Reliability and safety profile of long-term clinical application.1997, *Coron Artery Dis* 8(1):33-8.

[41] Kumar K. Toth C. Nath RK. Verma AK et al. Improvement of limb circulation in peripheral vascular disease using epidural spinal cord stimulation: a prospective study. *Journal of Neurosurg.*1997, 86(4):662-9.

[42] Huber S, Vagilenti R, Midcap R. et al. Enchansed limb salvage for peripheral vascular diseasewith the use of spinal cord stimulation. *W V Med J* 1996, 92:89-91.

[43] Petrakis E. Sciacca V. Prospective study of transcutaneous oxygen tension (TcPO2) measurement in the testing period of spinal cord stimulation in diabetic patients with critical lower limb ischaemia. *Intern Angiol* 2000, 19(1):18-25.

[44] Dumoulin K, Devulder J, Castille F et.al. A psychoanalytic investigation to improve the success rate of spinal cord stimulation as a treatment for chronic failed back surgery syndrome. *Clin J Pain* 1996;12(1):43-9.

[45] Bell GK, Kidd D, North RB. Cost-effectiveness analysis of spinal cord stimulation in treatment of failed back surgery syndrome. *J Pain Symptom Manage* 1997, 13(5):286-95.

[46] Bartolat G. A prospective multicenter study to assess the efficacy of spinal cord stimulation utilizing multi-channel radio-frequency system for the treatment of intractable low back pain and lower extremity pain. Initial considerations and methodology. *Neuromodulation* 1999,(2-3):179-183.

[47] Villavicencio AT. Leveque JC. Rubin L.et al. Laminectomy versus percutaneous electrode placement for spinal cord stimulation. *Neurosurg* 2000; 46(2):399-405, discussion 405-6.

In Frontiers in Pain Research
Editor: Alexendre Lucas, pp.113-132
ISBN 1-59454-828-5

Chapter 6

PAIN AND NEUROPLASTICITY IN HUMANS: CONTRIBUTION FROM NEUROPHYSIOLOGICAL STUDIES

Michele Tinazzi,* Paolo Invernizzi and Claudia Del Vesco
Dipartimento di Scienze Neurologiche e della Visione,
Sezione di Neurologia Riabilitativa, Università di Verona,
UO Neurologia Ospedale Civile Borgo Trento, Verona Italy

ABSTRACT

Studies in animals have shown that cortical representations of sensory surfaces reorganize after peripheral deafferentation so that some of the deprived cortex comes to be activated by inputs from skin regions near the deafferented zone. These changes may occur rapidly (short-term changes) or they may become progressively more pronounced over time (long-term changes). These changes of receptive fields are not confined to the cortex but also occur in the spinal dorsal horn and brainstem structures of the somatosensory system (for example in the cuneatus nucleus). Changes in subcortical structures could be one of the mechanisms subserving large scale reorganization in primary somatosensory cortex (S1). In humans, neurophysiologic techniques including magnetoencefalography (MEG), somatosensory evoked potentials (SEPs) and laser evoked potentials (LEPs) have been used to demonstrate aspects of short-tem and long-terms changes in the S1 and in subcortical structures in different conditions: i) in subjects after peripheral acute or chronic deafferentation; ii) in amputee patients with phantom limb pain and non-painful sensations; iii) in patients with chronic pain without massive large-fibres deafferentation; iiii) in normal subjects in whom pain was induced experimentally.

* Correspondence should be addressed to: Prof. Michele Tinazzi at: Dipartimento di Scienze Neurologiche e della Visione, Sezione di Neurologia Riabilitativa, Policlinico "G. B. Rossi", P.le A. L. Scuro, 37134, Verona. Voice: +39 45 8072601, Fax: +39 45 8072100, e-mail: michele.tinazzi@mail.azosp.vr.it

All these studies lead to the conclusion that pathological perturbations of somatic input may induce major neuroplastic changes at different levels of the Central Nervous System in humans and that pain is crucial in promoting reorganization in both somatosensory and nociceptive systems.

Key words: Pain; Neuroplasticity; Primary Somatosensory Cortex; Deafferentation.

INTRODUCTION

Convergent evidences from research in animals and humans indicate that physiological or pathological perturbations of somatic input may induce major neuroplastic changes at different levels of the somatosensory system even in adults (Jones, 2000). These changes may occur rapidly (short-term changes) (Merzenich et al. 1983b, Calford and Tweedale 1991) or the may become progressively more pronounced over time (long-term changes) (Merzenich et al. 1983 a, b). Short-term changes have been interpreted as reflecting an immediate unmasking (disinhibition) of pre-existing thalamocortical projections arising from skin territories adjacent to the deprived region (Merzenich et al. 1983b, Calford and Tweedale 1991; Garraghty et al. 1991; Schroeder et al. 1995). Long-term changes have been interpreted as reflecting increases in synaptic efficacy of previously existing synapses and also establishment of new anatomical connections (sprouting) (Merzenich et al. 1983 a,b; Raisman and Field 1988; Garraghty and Kaas 1991; Pons et al. 1991; Garraghty and Muja 1996). These changes have been documented by using two main approaches.

The first approach includes models in which neural changes are observed as consequence of an increase of sensory input. In animals, learning of tactile discrimination tasks or behaviour controlled tactile stimulation, brings about an increase of the neural representation in the primary somatosensory cortex (S1) of the skin surfaces engaged in the task (Jenkins *et al.*, 1990; Recanzone *et al.*, 1992b; Wang *et al.*, 1995). This remapping processes may have to do in humans with the enhancement of cortical activity evoked by stimulating the reading finger in Braille patients (Pascal-Leone and Torres 1993) or with the finger of the left hand in string players (Elbert et al. 1995). This "use-dependent" plasticity is typically beneficial (functionally relevant), because it is associated to a functional gain in perceptual sensory experiences.

The second approach includes models in which neural changes are observed as a consequence of decrease of sensory input: 1) functional decrease or 2) removal of afferent inputs (Kaas 2000). In the first condition, decreased use and reduced sensory feedback from a body part brings about a decrease of the neural representation in the S1 of the skin surfaces engaged in the task (Coq and Xerri, 1999; Langlet et al. 1999). In the second condition, it has been observed in animals that, after removal of afferent inputs, cortical territories formerly mapping the deafferented skin regions are driven by inputs coming from adjacent intact regions (Merzenich et al. 1983a,b; Pons et al. 1991; Florence and Kaas 1995). Short- and long-term reorganizations of receptive fields after peripheral deafferentation are not confined to the cortex but also occur in the spinal dorsal horn and brainstem structures of the somatosensory cortex (for example in the cuneatus nucleus) (Pettit and Schwark 1993; Florence and Kaas 1995; Faggin et al. 1997; Jain et al. 2000; Florence et al. 2000). Changes in subcortical structures could be one of the mechanisms subserving large scale reorganization in S1.

Functional neuroimaging as well as neurophysiology studies including magnetoencefalography (MEG) and somatosensory evoked potentials (SEPs), have provided evidence for remapping processes contingent upon a removal of somatosensory input in subjects with short- or long-lasting peripheral deafferentation (Rossini *et al.*, 1996; Tinazzi *et al.*, 1997; Tinazzi *et al.*, 1998) and in amputee humans (Elbert *et al.*, 1994; Yang et al. 1994; Flor et al. 1995, 1998; Grusser et al. 2001; Karl et al. 2001, 2004). This deafferentation-dependent plasticity is not functionally relevant. Instead, under some conditions, especially when pain coexists with massive deafferentation as in amputees patients with phantom pain limb, may be potentially maladaptative (Flor et al. 1995, 1998; Birbaumer et al. 1997; Grusser et al. 2001). Recently, plastic changes of somatic representation has been reported also in patients with chronic pain without large-diameter fibres deafferentation, as in low back pain, in cervical radiculopathy and in trigeminal neuralgia thus suggesting that ongoing pain stimulation per se may play an important role in determining rearrangements within the somatosensory system (Flor et al. 1997; Tinazzi et al. 2000, 2004). Finally, rapid changes in the nociceptive system have been demonstrated using the recording of laser evoked potentials (LEPs) in normal subjects in whom pain was induced experimentally (Valeriani et al. 2003, 2004). These findings suggest that pain *per se* may induce neuroplastic changes of somatic and nociceptive inputs within the Central Nervous System. In this chapter, we focus neurophysiological studies that deal with the interaction between nociceptive/non-nociceptive inputs and somatosensory/nociceptive systems and we discuss the possible relationship between pain and neuroplasticity.

NEUROPHYSIOLOGICAL STUDIES

MEG, SEPs and LEPs are neurophysiological non-invasive techniques which allow to assess the functional state of the somatosensory and nociceptive systems. The advantage of these techniques with respect of neuroimaging techniques including positron emission tomography (PET) and functional magnetic resonance imaging (fMRI) is that they allow to evaluate the time-course of excitatory and inhibitory effects within the somatosensory and nociceptive system. Indeed, neuroimaging techniques detect the total regional metabolism - the regional cerebral blood flow (rCBF) with PET and the blood oxygen level dependent (BOLD) signal with fMRI – and thus only give an indirect measure of neural activity without establishing if these changes refer to changes in excitatory and/or inhibitory neural activity. Moreover, these techniques only provide a steady-state picture of the phenomena, but the time course of the nociceptive-nonnociceptive interactions cannot be determined with a high temporal resolution.

Neurophysiological techniques have proved very useful in studying neuroplasticity in the human Central Nervous System showing aspects of short-tem and long terms changes in the S1 and in subcortical structures in different conditions: i) in subjects after peripheral acute or chronic deafferentation; ii) in amputee patients with phantom limb pain and non-painful sensations; iii) in patients with chronic pain without massive large-fibres deafferentation; iiii) in normal subjects in whom pain was induced experimentally.

Neuroplasticity Following Acute and Chronic Peripheral Deafferentation

Animal studies have shown that the cerebral cortex is capable of modification after partial peripheral deafferentation so that cortical territories formerly mapping the deafferented skin regions are driven by inputs coming from adjacent intact regions (Merzenich et al. 1983a, b; Calford and Tweedale 1991; Pons et al. 1991). These changes may occur rapidly (short-term changes) (Merzenich et al. 1983b; Calford and Tweedale 1991) and, depending on the type of deafferentation (transient or permanent) may be reversible or progressively develop over time (long-term changes) (Merzenich et al. 1983a,b). It has been demonstrated that short and long-term receptive fields reorganization is not restricted to the cerebral cortex but also occurs in the spinal dorsal-horn and brainstem structures which could be responsible for most of the cortical large-scale S1 reorganization (Pettit and Schwark 1993; Florence and Kaas 1995; Faggin et al. 1997; Jain et al. 2000; Florence et al. 2000). Such phenomena have been replicated in humans in both acute and chronic conditions of peripheral deafferentation (Rossini et al. 1994; Tinazzi et al. 1997, 1998).

Using MEG, Rossini et al. (1994) firstly reported in normal subjects the effect of a transient peripheral deafferentation of the fingers on cortical S1 reorganization. Somatosensory Evoked Fields (SEFs) were recorded during separate electrical stimulation of the 1st, 3rd, or 5th finger before, during and after an anaesthetic block (obtained with lidocaine) of the four non-stimulated fingers. It was observed that the SEFs responsible for the cortical responses from the unanaesthetized finger were significantly changed following a relatively brief period of sensory deprivation from the adjacent fingers. Such SEFs changes were characterized by an increase in strength and deepening for the middle finger, and by a shift on the coronal plane for the thumb and the little finger (medial for the former, lateral for the latter) during anaesthesia and persisted for several minutes after the anaesthesia disappeared. This cortical modulation has been interpreted to reflect immediate unmasking of pre-existing but physiologically "inactive" thalamo-cortical projections from skin territories adjacent to deafferented zone (Calford and Tweedale 1991; Merzenich et 1983b; Schroeder et al. 1995). This mechanism has been hypothesized to be mediated by a decrease of intracortical gamma-aminobutyric acid (GABA) inhibition, since intracortical administration of a GABA antagonist induced a similar modulation of the cortical map (Jacobs and Donoghue 1991) and since injury-induced S1 reorganization was accompanied by reductions in GABA staining (Garraghty et al. 1990). In this respect, short-term changes of SEFs have been suggested to reflect disinhibition of latent thalamo-cortical projections arising from fingers cutaneous territories adjacent to the anaesthetized finger. The same mechanism has been assumed to explain the increase in rCBF in the sensori-motor cortex after temporary deafferentation of forearm (Sadato et al. 1995). Nevertheless an important question is if these rapid plastic changes are specifically related to the cortex or if they indicate changes in neural activity in the dorsal horn or the nucleus cuneatus.

This issue was addressed by Tinazzi et al. (1997) by recording SEPs obtained by stimulation of the median nerve before, during and after anaesthetic block of the ipsilateral ulnar nerve. Unlike MEG, SEPs recording allows to assess spinal, brainstem and cortical neural activity of the lemniscal pathway. This may be important to establish if cortical changes are possibly dependent on subcortical changes.

Amplitudes of spinal N13 and P14 potentials, reflecting the post-synaptic neuronal activity of the dorsal horn and of the cuneatus nucleus respectively (Desmedt and Cheron

1980; Zanette et al. 1995), remained unchanged during the experiment, while cortical SEPs increased in amplitude during the anaesthetic block and then returned to the baseline values 20 minutes after the end of the anaesthetic period. The Authors concluded that these rapid changes in S1 cortical excitability occur independently on changes in the lowest structures of the somatosensory system. These findings seem inconsistent with animal studies which have shown that in spinal cord dorsal horn and nucleus cuneatus, as in the cortex, receptive fields may also rapidly reorganize after peripheral denervation and local anaethesia by nerve injections, although this reorganization is typically more limited in extent than that in S1 (Dostrovsky et al. 1976; Pettit and Schwark 1993). One possible explanation of this discrepancy may be due that changes in receptive fields observed from single or small populations of neurons are not directly comparable with SEPs which are recorded far from their putative generators and represent synchronized activity of neurons. Moreover, averaging of 500 responses which is necessary to record reliable SEPs may attenuate changes in neural excitability occurring within several minutes with the result that limited neural changes may be masked. So, the immediate and transient modulation of the S1 excitability we have observed (Tinazzi et al. 1997) appeared not related to spinal and brainstem modulation, at least in the experimental conditions under which are recorded SEPs. Thus, modulation of S1 excitability might be due mainly to changes in the excitability of the intracortical network. An interesting finding from this study was that S1 modulation appeared to occur independently and to a variable degree within the different subareas of S1, because of the different behaviours of the N20/P20, P27 and N30 potentials. The N20/P20 and N30 potentials which are generated in area 3b presented the greatest and more constant amplitude changes during the anaesthetic block (Allison et al. 1991). Minimal and variable changes were observed for P27 potential, which is generated in area 1 (Allison et al. 1991). These findings may agree with experimental data obtained in animal models where receptive fields reorganization was found to be more marked in area 3b than in area 1 (Merzenich et al. 1983a, b).

All these data have suggested that short-term changes in the neural activity of the human S1 following transient peripheral deafferentation seem mostly independent on changes in excitability at subcortical levels and that these changes are segregated in the different subareas of S1.

Studies from animals have shown that short-term changes that follow peripheral nerve transection account for only a small minority of the changes in the cortical topography occurring over weeks or months. Aspects of this long-term modulation in the human somatosensory system have been provided by a study of our group (Tinazzi et al. 1998). We have assessed spinal, brainstem and cortical SEPs obtained to stimulation of the ulnar nerve in patients affected by unilateral carpal syndrome without pain, who had EMG evidence of chronic abnormality of median nerve sensorimotor conduction at the wrist lasting at least 4 week and compared them with those from the unaffected hand and with those obtained in a control group. Amplitudes of spinal and brainstem components following stimulation of the ulnar nerve ipsilateral to the deafferented median nerve were greater than those following stimulation of the contralateral ulnar nerve. Side-to-side amplitude differences in N13 and P14 were greater in patients than in the control group. Cortical components originating in S1 were also significantly increased in amplitude. We concluded that this long-term S1 modulation might be related to changes in spinal and brainstem structures while short-term S1 modulation is not. The thalamus may also contribute to this modulation as documented in animals (Nicolelis et al. 1993). Unfortunatly, there is no reliable evidence that specific SEP responses reflecting neural activity of the ventroposterolateral thalamic nucleus can be recorded over the scalp. In animals, median nerve transection is followed by a predictable sequence of changes within the deprived portion of the somatosensory structures which probably occurs in two phases (Merzenich et al. 1983a, b; Garraghty et al. 1990; Garraghty and Kaas 1991; Calford and Tweedale 1991; Garraghty and Muja 1996; Schroeder et al 1995). In the first phase, some deprived neurons immediately express new receptive fields, while in the second phase the remaining neurons regain responsiveness over the ensuing weeks or months. The initial phase (described above) is probably due to unmasking of pre-existing thalamocortical projections and it seems GABA-mediated (Garraghty et al. 1990; Jacobs and Donoghue 199), while the second phase, which probably is mediated by NMDA receptors (Garraghty and Muja 1996) is characterized by more pronounced topographic changes (normally completed in 4 weeks) which have been interpreted as reflecting a gradual synaptic strengthening secondary to the disconnection of the normally dominant inputs to the "median nerve" cortex (Merzenich et al. 1983a, b; Garraghty and Kaas 1991; Garraghty and Muja 1996). Sprouting processes may also contribute to long-term changes. These mechanisms have been claimed to explain the increase in SEP responses in patients with carpal tunnel syndrome. Similar mechanisms have been assumed to explain the increase in regional CBF and rearrangement of magnetic fields in S1 in long-standing amputee patients (Elbert et al. 1994; Yang et al. 1994; Kew et al. 1994; Flor et al. 1995)

Whatever the precise mechanisms, changes in ulnar SEPs were not related to any sensory perceptual advantage for the patients in the ulnar nerve skin regions ipsilateral to the deafferented median nerve. Gains in perceptual sensory experience of a body part secondary to increased use and enhanced sensory feedback of that body part are usually regarded as an indicator of progressive S1 modulation (Jenkins et al. 1990; Recanzone et al. 1992 a, b, c, d; Wang et al. 1995). It is therefore plausible that the increase in ulnar nerve SEPs was not due to an enhanced sensory feedback from the ulnar nerve skin regions but was rather due to the removal of normally dominant inputs from the ipsilateral median nerve. These findings suggest that neuroplasticity following chronic deafferentation are not functionally relevant for the subject.

Neuroplasticity in Amputee Patients with Phantom Limb Pain and Non-Painful Sensations

Several evidences indicate that, under some conditions, especially when pain coexists with massive large-fibres deafferentation, neuroplasticity may be potentially maladaptative.

In animals peripheral neurectomy or dorsal rhizotomy (in rodents) is followed by self-mutilation in which the animals bite and scratch the insensate paw to the point. This behaviour is produced by ongoing pain or disesthesia and is associated to plastic changes in the CNS. In amputee patients it has been firstly assumed (Katz 1992) that cortical reorganization might be an adaptative process that protects the amputee from the development of phantom limb pain. Contrary to this assumption, Flor et al. (1995) reported a high positive correlation between the magnitude of phantom limb pain and the amount of cortical reorganization which is consistent with Melzack's assumption of a "neuromatrix" underlying phantom limb pain. This suggests that cortical reorganization in response to amputation may be potentially maladaptative. According to several surveys phantom limb sensations are reported by 70-100% of amputees, and phantom limb pain occurs in 50-80 % of these cases (Kooijman et al. 2000; Sherman 1989; Wartan et al. 1997). Nevertheless, phantom limb sensations and phantom limb pain have different relationship with cortical reorganization. Ramachandram et al. (1992) observed in three amputees that light touches with a cotton swab or deep pressure to either the face or the stump would often elicit referred sensation in the phantom, sometimes with a point-to-point correspondence of stimulation sites and locations of referred sensation in the phantom. These anomalous double sensations evoked by tactile stimulation of intact skin regions have been reported not only in limb amputees but also in breast amputees, and more recently in patients with a lesion of the primary somatosensory cortex (Aglioti et al.1994 a, b, 1997; Halligan et al. 1994; Knecht et al. 1998; Aglioti et al. 1999). Ramachandran et al. (1992b) suggested that this phenomenon might be the perceptual correlate of cortical reorganization occurring subsequent to amputation. However recent MEG studies have documented that cortical reorganization is not related to the presence of referred sensations but rather highly positively correlated with the magnitude of phantom limb pain experienced by the subjects but not with non-painful phantom sensations (Elbert et al. 1994; Flor et al. 1995, 1998, 2000; Knecth et al. 1996; Birbaumer et al. 1997; Borsook et al. 1998; Montoya et al. 1998; Grusser et al. 2001). Functional neuroimaging studies have revealed a similar positive correlation between pain and reorganization of sensori-motor cortex (Kew et al. 1994, 1997; Lotze et al. 1999; Willoch et al. 2000). In MEG studies while amputees with phantom limb pain showed an average cortical reorganization in the range of 1-2 cm, pain-free amputees showed only marginal changes. However, further examination revealed that non-painful phantom sensations such as referred sensations and telescoping arm are related to changes in the posterior and /or secondary somatosensory cortex.

Knecht et al. (1998) assessed shifts of representational zones by magnetic source imaging in 8 arm-amputee patients and examined them for referred sensation by somaesthetic stimuli of different modalities at standardized sites. It was found that referred phantom sensations could be evoked from sites on the face and the trunk ipsilateral but also controlateral to the amputation and that the extent of physiological reorganization as revealed by magnetic source imaging strongly correlates with the number of sites, being them ipsi- or controlateral, from where painful stimuli evoke referred sensation. Thus, it seems that the extent of reorganization after amputation is closely related to nociceptive inputs. The mislocalization evoked from both sides of the body, suggesting involvement of bilateral pathways, demonstrated that the perceptual changes go beyond what can be explained by shifts in neighbouring cortical representational zones.

Flor et al. (1998) using MEG, assessed, the relationship between phantom limb phenomena and cortical reorganization in five subjects with congenital absence of an upper limb and nine traumatic amputees. The purpose of the study was to carry out a detailed analysis of the organization of the SI by neuromagnetic source imaging and to determine its relationship with both painful and nonpainful phantom phenomena in congenital and traumatic amputees. The study shows that in accordance with the absence of phantom phenomena, cortical reorganization in the congenital amputees was low and not significantly different from that of traumatic amputees without phantom limb pain. In contrast , traumatic amputees with phantom limb pain showed substantial cortical reorganization, as previously reported.

Similarly, Montoya et al. (1998) tested with MEG the extent of the cortical somatotopic map and its relationship to phantom phenomena in five subjects with congenital absence of an upper limb, four traumatic amputees with phantom limb pain and five healty controls. Cortical map of the first and fifth digit of the intact hand, the lower lip and the first toe were obtained using neuroelectric source imaging. The subjects with congenital upper limb atrophy showed symmetric positions of the left and right side of the lower lip and the first toe, whereas the traumatic amputees with pain showed a significant shift of the cortical representation of the lower lip towards the hand region contralateral to the amputation side but no shift for the toe representation. Phantom phenomena were absent in the congenital but extensive in the traumatic amputees. These data confirmed the assumption that congenital absence of a limb does not lead to cortical reorganization or phantom limb, whereas traumatic amputations, that are accompanied by phantom limb pain, show shifts of the cortical areas adjacent to the amputations zone towards the representation of the deafferented body part. These neurophysiological observations are consistent with PET and fMRI studies performed in congenital upper limb amputees and in patients with acquired amputation presenting or not phantom limb symptoms. Kew et al. (1994) demonstrated with PET a greater metabolic activity in S1-M1 during limb movements in patients with acquired amputation with phantom limb pain than in patients with congenital amputation. In addition they observed (Kew et al. 1997) in two patients with complete deafferentation of one upper limb secondary to traumatic multiple cervical root avulsions that vibrotactile stimulation of the skin in the pectoral region ipsilateral to the amputation eliciting referred sensation in the phantom limb was associated with activation of the controlateral S1 that extended ventrally from the level of the trunk representation. This suggests that sensory inputs delivered to the axial body surface may gain access to the S1 hand/arm area in some humans who have suffered extensive deafferentation of this area. More recently, Willoch et al (2000) used PET to study phantom limb pain and other phantom limb sensations. To induce these phenomena they used hypnosis. So, they induced in human amputees phantom sensations of comfortable position, comfortable movement, painful position and painful movement and observed different cortical activation through PET. During comfortable movement they observed activation of SM1 and SMA controlateral area. During painful movement they observed also activation of the insula, the anterior cingulate cortex and the prefrontal cortex in an area covering parts of the inferior an middle frontal gyri. During painful posture they observed activation of controlateral SM1, SMA, controlateral anterior cingulate cortex, left prefrontal cortex (inferior frontal gyrus), the controlateral lenticular nucleus and the thalamus. The greatest difference between comfortable movement and painful position activation was in the anterior cingulate cortex and in the thalamus. Both of them are considered fundamental elements in the normal circuitry processing pain and are part of the medial pain system (cingulate gyrus, insula, lateral prefrontal cortex and anteromedially lying intralaminar thalamic nuclei) concerned with the emotional and motivational processing of pain. So, the results provided evidence that phantom limb experiences are produced by the same brain processes that underlie the experience of the body when it is intact and that phantom limb pain is associated with propagation of activity in a thalamocortical network normally processing externally applied or modulated pain.

In amputees with or without plantom limb pain, Lotze et al (2001) studied brain activation (through fMRI) during hand and lip movement and imagined movements of the phantom limb. Lip movement ipsilateral to the amputation side revealed a shift of the medial border of the cortical rappresentation in both M1 and S1 areas into the deafferented hand area only in subjects suffering phantom limb pain; this difference was not significant for patients with non-painful phantom limb phenomena. So, it is evident that cortical reorganization in M1/S1 controlateral to amputation is correlated with the experience of phantom limb pain and the pain experience seems to modulate reorganization in cortical area via thalamocortical pathways.

All these data indicate that phantom limb pain rather phantom limb sensations is related to plastic changes in sensori-motor cortex.

A strong functional link between cortical reorganization and phantom limb pain is also suggested by the fact that suppressing phantom pain brought about a clear reduction of cortical reorganization of the ipsilateral lower lip (Birbaumer et al., 1997). Brachial plexus anaesthesia has been used to eliminate peripheral input to the amputation and to further evaluate the relationship of cortical reorganization and phantom limb pain stump. In about half of the amputee sample studied, brachial plexus anesthesia eliminated phantom limb pain, in the other half of the sample phantom limb remained unchanged. EEG-based source imaging of S1 revealed that the reduction in phantom limb pain was mirrored by a reversal of cortical reorganization, whereas amputees without pain-reduction showed increased cortical reorganization due to the anesthesia-induced loss of input from the periphery. These data suggest that there is a functional relationship between cortical reorganization and phantom limb pain. It is unlikely, however that cortical reorganization maintains phantom limb pain by itself: removal of portions of postcentral gyrus does not always successfully abolish phantom limb pain (Kenshalo and Douglas 1995) and subcortical structures may also play an important role (Florence and Kaas 1995; Faggin et al. 1997; Jones 2000; Jain et al. 2000; Florence et al. 2000).

Neuroplasticity in Patients with Chronic Pain without Large-Fibres Deafferentation

In the above studies pain coexisted with large-diameter fibres deafferentation that is known to promote neuroplastic changes per se (Florence and Kaas 1995; Tinazzi et al. 1997; 1998). However, animal and human studies suggest that ongoing pain stimulation per se may play an important role in determining cortical rearrangements also in absence of large-diameter fibres deafferentation and may contribute to the persistence of the experience of pain.

In animals it has been demonstrated that intense noxious stimulation or tissue injury can produce dramatic changes in the sensitivity to both noxius and non-noxius stimulation as well as expansion of the receptive fields of neurones of the dorsal horn (Perl 1976; Price et al. 1978; Kensalo et al. 1979, 1982; Simone et al. 1991; Dougherty and Willis 1992), thalamus (Guilbaud et al. 1986) and somatosensory cortex (Lamour et al. 1983).

Evidence in humans come from studies in patients with low back pain, in patients with cervical radicular pain and in patients with trigeminal neuralgia (Flor et al. 1997; Tinazzi et al. 2000, 2004). In patients with low-back pain, Flor et al. (1997) demonstrated an expansion of the cortical representation of the back in a more medial direction (toward the foot area). It has been assumed that this expansion might be related to ongoing noxious input emanating from the affected body region since the hand representation was unaltered. The enhanced activity related to back stimulation was positively correlated with the duration of the pain. In a similar vein, we have demonstrated using the SEPs recording technique, plastic changes at multiple levels of the somatosensory system in patients with cervical radicular pain (Tinazzi et al. 2000). These patients complained of pain to the right thumb following a right cervical monoradiculopathy due to compression of the sixth cervical root, in spite of any clinico-neurophysiological signs of large-fibres deafferentation. We found that amplitudes of spinal, brainstem and cortical SEPs to stimulation of the patients' right painful thumb were greater than those recorded in response to stimulation of the non-painful left thumb and those recorded in controls. This left-right difference in amplitude was not observed following stimulation of the non-painful third fingers. Thus, the increased excitability of spinal, brainstem and cortical structures was specific to the painful region.

The absence of correlation between the amplitudes of spinal, brainstem and cortical components of SEPs suggested that enhancement of cortical activity is not a simple amplification of subcortical enhancement. In keeping with the study of Flor et al. (1997) in patients with chronic low back pain, we failed to find any correlation between central SEPs evoked by stimulation of the painful thumb and measures of sensitivity to pain in the same region. This lack of relationship, however, may suggest that the SEP technique is sensitive enough to detect pathophysiological modifications before the appearence of clinical symptoms.

By contrast, a significant, positive correlation between amplitudes of central SEPs to stimulation of the painful thumb and magnitude of subjective measures of pain intensity was detected, thus suggesting that the increased amplitude of central SEPs reported above can be attributed to pain *per se*. These observations suggest that ongoing pain stimulation per se, in absence of large-diameter fibres deafferentation, may lead to an enlargement of the cortical representation and an increased neural reactivity to somatic inputs input coming from the same painful skin territory (Floor et al. 1997; Tinazzi et al. 2000). This suggested that plastic changes can occur across different somatic submodalities (nociceptive and cutaneous) subserving the same cutaneous territory (Tinazzi et al. 2004), a finding that is consistent with evidence of plastic changes across other submodalities, i.e. cutaneous and proprioceptive submodalities (Xerri et al. 1999; Tinazzi et al. 2003).

Recent studies indicate that pain per se may also induce neuroplastic changes of somatic inputs coming from cutaneous territories with contiguous neural representation. Tinazzi et al. (2004) assessed SEPs in patients with idiopathic right unilateral trigeminal neuralgia, a disorder of the fifth cranial (trigeminal) nerve that causes episodes of intense, stabbing electric shock-like pain in areas of the face where the nerve branches are distributed. It is worth noting that paroxysmal pain in idiopathic trigeminal neuralgia seems to be primarily related to a dysfunction of Adelta afferents althoug minor involvement of myelinic Abeta fibers has been demonstrated (Cruccu et al. 1990; 2001; 2002). We found that cortical SEPs obtained from the median nerve ipsilateral to facial pain localized to the mandibular/maxillary branch of the nerve were greater than those obtained from the contralateral hand and these changes were related to pain experienced by patients. No side-to-side asymmetry was found in amplitude of potentials evoked by stimulation of the tibial nerve. Given the representational contiguity of face and hand in the somatosensory cortex, this suggests that pain-related somatic changes can occur across representations mapping different somatic inputs coming from adjacent skin territories. These results added to the body evidence pointing to the important role of pain in inducing neuroplastic effects across channels dedicated to different somatic modalities as touch (Birbaumer et al. 1997; Flor et al. 1995, 1997; Juottonen et al. 2002; Tinazzi et al. 2000; Rosso et al. 2003).

These results are also in keeping with a recent behavioural study reporting that acute pain *per se* may induce mislocation phenomena even in intact humans (Knecht et al., 1998). These authors applied acute pain to the hand followed by non-noxious tactile stimulation of the ipsilateral lip and serendipitously found that subjects reported phantom like sensations on the hand synchronous to the lip stimulation. This has been interpreted as the perceptual correlate of unmasked silent connections between neural regions mapping hand and lip. In view of this result we assessed whether tactile stimulation of the hand could elicit double sensations on the face (Tinazzi et al. 2004). No phantom pain or tactile sensations were elicited in patients with trigeminal neuralgia. Although speculative, a possible explanation for this is that patients were not tested during episodes of paroxysmal pain..

Neuroplasticity Following Pain Induced Experimentally

Recently, plastic changes of somatic representation induced by pain has been also reported in an experimental model of nociceptive pain in which acute pain was induced by intradermal injection of capsaicin in the hand of normal subjects (Soros et al. 2001). The Authors observed that pain was associated with changes of MEG components evoked by tactile stimulation of the lower lip ipsilateral to the injected hand (Soros et al. 2001) characterized by a decrease of distance between cortical and hand representation. They concluded that this modulation induced by pain lead to hyperresponsiveness to tactile input from neighboring body site and that it may be the neurophysiological correlates of mislocation phenomena observed in normal subjects after induction of acute pain (Knetch et al. 1998).

Recently Valeriani et al. (2003, 2004) have demonstrated that acute pain in normal subjects may induce neuroplastic changes not only in the lemniscal pathwhay but also in the nociceptive system. In the first study they assessed the effect of acute pain induced by capsaicin in cerebral areas devoted to nociceptive input processing through Laser-Evoked Potentials (LEPs). CO_2 stimulation of the skin offers the opportunity to selectively stimulate nociceptive afferents (A delta and C afferents) without any concurrent stimulation of cutaneous or proprioceptive afferents. LEPs were recorded from 10 healthy subjects before and 20-30 minutes after capsaicin application over the dorsum of the hand and finally 10-20 minutes after capsaicin removal. LEPs were significantly decreased in amplitude during capsaicin and after capsaicin removal. Moreover, the topography of the vertex LEP components was modified after capsaicin removal, moving from the central toward the parietal region. Dipolar modelling showed that dipolar source in the anterior cingulate cortex, which generates the vertex LEP components, moved backward after capsaicin removal. These changes were not observed after stimulation of hand controlateral to the induced pain, thus suggesting that functional changes are selective for the painful skin and adjacent skin territories. This indicated that painful stimuli delivered to a given nociceptive channel bring about a decrease in activity in adjacent nociceptive channels. The Authors concluded that acute cutaneous pain induces a short- term inhibition of the cingulated cortex, which generates the N2a- P2 potential . Therefore, the role of cingulated cortex inhibition due to acute pain could be addressed to reduce the emotional and affective aspects of noxious stimuli delivered within or near a painful skin area.

Moreover, Valeriani et al. (2004) evaluated the effect of tonic pain evoked by topical application of capsaicin on the somatosensory sensation of warmth. The warmth pathways were studied in healthy subjects by recording the scalp potentials evoked by non-painful warm laser stimuli delivered on both the right and left perioral region (warmth C-fiber related laser-evoked potentials (C-LEPs)). Tonic pain was induced by topical capsaicin application above the lateral part of the right upper lip. The area of primary and secondary hyperalgesia were mapped. C-LEPs were obtained before, during, and after capsaicin application. C-LEPs from the right perioral region were evoked by laser stimuli delivered to the area of secondary hyperalgesia during capsaicin application and on both the areas of primary and secondary hyperalgesia after capsaicin removal. While the lateralized N1/P1 component (around 185 ms of latency which is originated in the SII) was not affected by the capsaicin, the amplitudes of the later vertex C-LEPs (around 260 and 410 ms of latency for the N2a and P2 potentials respectively, which are generated in the anterior cingulate cortex) evoked from the secondary hyperalgesic area on the right side and from a symmetrical non-hyperalgesic area on the left perioral region were significantly decreased during capsaicin application and after capsaicin removal, as compared with the baseline recordings. At the same times, the rating of the laser-evoked warmth sensation was reduced significantly. This inhibitory effect can occur at brainstem level via trigemino-cortico-trigeminal circuits, similar to those mediating the classical diffuse noxious inhibitory control. Probably due to a peripheral inhibitory mechanism, neither reliable C-LEP components nor warmth sensation were evoked by laser pulses delivered to the primary hyperalgesic area. The Authors concluded that the inhibitory effect of pain on warmth sensation as revealed by a decrease of N2a/P2 components may have the functional meaning of reduce the affective and emotional aspect of warmth. These observations are consistent with previous functional neuroimaging studies (Iadarola et al. 1998; Olausson et al. 2001; Peyron et al. 2000; Casey et al. 1994, 1996; Svensson et al. 1997; Talbot et al. 1991; Coghill et al. 1994) showing that acute pain in humans may induce neuroplastic changes within the nociceptive system.

Conclusion

All these studies provide evidence of heavy interactions in the CNS between nociceptive/non-nociceptive afferents that are involved in the neuroplasticity of the somatosensory/nociceptive systems induced by deafferentation. This form of plasticity is not benefical for the subjects but instead may be maladaptative because it may represent the perceptual correlate of pain and other pain symptoms such as allodinia or hyperalgesia. Further studies should be addressed to understand the precise mechanisms leading to this plasticity in order to design effective, rational pharmacological and rehabilitative therapeutic strategies to down regulating this maladaptative plasticity thus promoting the recovery of function.

REFERENCES

Aglioti S, Bonazzi A, Cortese F. Phantom lower limb as a perceptual marker of neural plasticity in the mature human brain. *Proc Biol Sci.* 1994 Mar 22;255(1344):273-8.

Aglioti S, Smania N, Atzei A, Berlucchi G. Spatio-temporal properties of the pattern of evoked phantom sensations in a left index amputee patient. *Behav Neurosci.* 1997 Oct;111(5):867-72.

Aglioti S, Beltramello A, Peru A, Smania N, Tinazzi M. Anomalous double sensations after damage to the cortical somatosensory representation of the hand in humans.*Neurocase* 1999 Vol.5 pp 285-292.

Allison T, McCarthy G, Wood CC, Jones SJ. Potentials evoked in human and monkey cerebral cortex by stimulation of the median nerve. A review of scalp and intracranial recordings.*Brain.* 1991 Dec;114 (Pt 6):2465-503.

Allison T, Wood CC, McCarthy G, Spencer DD. Cortical somatosensory evoked potentials. II. Effects of excision of somatosensory or motor cortex in humans and monkeys. J *Neurophysiol.* 1991 Jul;66(1):64-82.

Birbaumer N, Lutzenberger W, Montoya P, Larbig W, Unertl K, Topfner S, Grood W, Taub E, Flor H. Effects of regional anesthesia on phantom limb pain are mirrored in changes in cortical reorganization. *J Neurosci* 1997; Jul 15; 17: 5503-5508.

Borsook D, Becerra L, Fishman S, Edwards A, Jennings CL, Stojanovic M, Papinicolas L, Ramachandran VS, Gonzalez RG, Breiter H. Acute plasticity in the human somatosensory cortex following amputation. *Neuroreport.* 1998 Apr 20;9(6):1013-7.

Calford MB, Tweedale R. Acute changes in cutaneous receptive fields in primary somatosensory cortex after digit denervation in adult flying fox. *J Neurophysiol.* 1991 Feb;65(2):178-87.

Calford MB, Tweedale R. Immediate expansion of receptive fields of neurons in area 3b of macaque monkeys after digit denervation. *Somatosens Mot Res.* 1991;8(3):249-60.

Carlen PL, Wall PD, Nadvorna H, Steinbach T. Phantom limbs and related phenomena in recent traumatic amputations. *Neurology* 1978 Mar; 28:211-217.

Casey KL, Minoshima S, Morrow TJ, Koeppe RA. Comparison of human cerebral activation patterns during cutaneous warmth, heat pain, and deep cold pain. *J of Neurophysiol* 1996 Jul; 76: 571-581.

Casey KL, Minoshima S, Berger KL, Koeppe RA, Morrow TJ, Frey KA. Positron emission tomographic analysis of cerebral structures activated specifically by repetetive noxious heat stimuli. *J Neurophysiol.* 1994 Feb; 71: 802-807.

Coghill RC, Talbot JD, Evans AC, Meyer E, Gjedde A, Bushnell MC, Duncan GH. Distributed processing of pain and vibration by the human brain. *J Neurosci.* 1994 Jul;14(7):4095-108.

Cohen LG, Bandinelli S, Findley TW, Hallett M. Motor reorganization after upper limb amputation in man (a study with focal magnetic stimulation). *Brain* 1991 Feb; 114: 615-627.

Coq O-J, Xerri C. Tactile impoverishment and sensorimotor restriction deteriorate the forepaw cutaneous map in the primary somatosensory cortex of adult rats. *Exp Brain Res* 1999 Dec; 129: 518-531.

Cruccu G, Leandri M, Feliciani M, Manfredi M. Idiopathic and symptomatic trigeminal pain. *J Neurol Neurosurg Psychiatry.* 1990 Dec;53(12):1034-42.

Cruccu G, Inghilleri M, Berardelli A, Pauletti G, Manfredi M. Cortico-facial and cortico-trigeminal projections. A comparison by magnetic brain stimulation in man. *Electroencephalogr Clin Neurophysiol Suppl.* 1990;41:140-4.

Cruccu G, Truini A, Priori A. Excitability of the human trigeminal motoneuronal pool and interactions with other brainstem reflex pathways. *J Physiol.* 2001 Mar 1;531(Pt 2):559-71.

Cruccu G, Galeotti F, Iannetti GD, Romaniello A, Truini A, Manfredi M. Trigeminal neuralgia: update on reflex and evoked potential studies. *Mov Disord.* 2002;17 Suppl 2:S37-40.

Desmedt JE, Cheron G. Central somatosensory conduction in man: neural generators and interpeak latencies of the far-field components recorded from neck and right or left scalp and earlobes.*Electroencephalogr Clin Neurophysiol.* 1980 Dec;50(5-6):382-403.

Desmedt JE, Nguyen TH, Bourguet M. Bit-mapped color imaging of human evoked potentials with reference to the N20, P22, P27 and N30 somatosensory responses. *Electroencephalogr Clin Neurophysiol.* 1987 Jan;68(1):1-19.

Dostrovsky JO, Millar J, Wall PD. The immediate shift of afferent drive of dorsal column nucleus cells following deafferentation: a comparison of acute and chronic deafferentation in gracile nucleus and spinal cord. *Exp Neurol* 1976 Sep; 52: 480-495.

Dougherty PM, Willis WD. Enhanced responses of spinothalamic tract neurons to excitatory amino acids accompany capsaicin-induced sensitization in the monkey. *J Neurosci.* 1992 Mar;12(3):883-94.

Elbert T, Flor H, Birbaumer N, Knecht S, Hampson S, Larbig W, Taub E. Extensive reorganisation of the somatosensory cortex in adult humans after nervous system injury. *Neuroreport* 1994 Dec; 5: 2593-2597.

Elbert T, Pantev C, Wienbruch C, Rockstroh B, Taub E. Increased cortical representation of the fingers of the left hand in string players. *Science* 1995 Oct; 270: 305-307.

Faggin BM, Nguyen KY, Nicolelis MA. Immediate and simultaneous sensory reorganisation at cortical and subcortical levels of the somatosensory system. Proc Natl Acad Sci USA 1997 Aug 19; 94: 9428-9433.

Flor H, Elbert T, Knecht S, Wienbruch C, Pantev C, Birbaumer N, et al. Phantom-limb as a perceptual correlate of cortical reorganisation following arm amputation. *Nature* 1995 Jun 8; 375: 482-484.

Flor H, Braun C, Elbert T, Birbaumer N. Extensive reorganization of primary somatosensory cortex in chronic back pain patients. *Neurosci Letters* 1997 Mar 7; 224: 5-8.

Flor H, Elbert T, Muhlnickel W, Pantev C, Wienbruch C, Taub E. Cortical reorganization and phantom phenomena in congenital and traumatic upper-extremity amputees. *Exp Brain Res.* 1998 Mar;119(2):205-12.

Flor H. [Helping patients with phantom pain. Prosthesis for the brain?. Interview by Dipl. Biochem. Petra Eiden.] *MMW Fortschr Med.* 1999 Dec 16;141(51-52):16.

Flor H, Muhlnickel W, Karl A, Denke C, Grusser S, Kurth R, Taub E. A neural substrate for non painful phantom limb phenomena. *Neuroreport.* 2000 May 15;11(7):1407-11.

Florence SL, Kaas JH. Large-scale reorganisation at multiple levels of the somatosensory pathway follows therapeutic amputation of the hand in monkeys. *J Neuroscience* 1995 Dec; 15: 8083-8095.

Florence SL, Hackett TA, Strata F. Thalamic and cortical contributions to neural plasticity after limb amputation. *J Neurophysiol.* 2000 May;83(5):3154-9.

Garraghty PE, Florence SL, Kaas JH Ablations of areas 3a and 3b of monkey somatosensory cortex abolish cutaneous responsivity in area 1. *Brain Res.* 1990 Sep 24;528(1):165-9.

Garraghty PE, Kaas JH. Functional reorganization in adult monkey thalamus after peripheral nerve injury. *Neuroreport.* 1991 Dec;2(12):747-50.

Garraghty PE, Kaas JH. Large-scale functional reorganization in adult monkey cortex after peripheral nerve injury. *Proc Natl Acad Sci U S A.* 1991 Aug 15;88(16):6976-80.

Garraghty PE, Muja N. NMDA receptors and plasticity in adult primate somatosensory cortex. *J Comp Neurol.* 1996 Apr 1;367(2):319-26.

Grusser SM, Winter C, Muhlnickel W, Denke C, Karl A, Villringer K, Flor H. The relationship of perceptual phenomena and cortical reorganization in upper extremity amputees. *Neuroscience.* 2001;102(2):263-72.

Grusser SM, Winter C, Schaefer M, Fritzsche K, Benhidjeb T, Tunn P, Schlag PM, Flor H. perceptual phenomena after unilateral arm amputation: a pre-post-surgical comparison. *Neurosci Lett.* 2001 Apr 13;302(1):13-6.

Grusser SM, Winter C, Muhlnickel W, Denke C, Karl A, Villringer K, Flor H. The relationship of perceptual phenomena and cortical reorganization in upper extremity amputees. *Neuroscience.* 2001;102(2):263-72.

Guilbaud G, Kaiser V, Benoist JM, Gautron M. Modifications in the responsiveness of rat ventrobasal thalamic neurons at different stages of carrageenin-produced inflammation. *Brain Res* 1986 Oct 15; 385: 86-98.

Halligan PW, Marshall JC, Wade DT. Sensory disorganization and perceptual plasticity after limb amputation: a follow-up study. *Neuroreport.* 1994 Jun 27;5(11):1341-5.

Iadarola MJ, Berman KF, Zeffiro TA, Byas-Smith MG, Gracely RH, Max MB, Bennett GJ. Neural activation during acute capsaicin-evoked pain and allodynia assessed with PET. *Brain.* 1998 May;121 (Pt 5):931-47.

Jacobs KM, Donoghue JP. Reshaping the cortical motor map by unmasking latent intracortical connections. *Science.* 1991 Feb 22;251(4996):944-7.

Jain N, Florence SL, Qi HX, Kaas JH. Growth of new brainstem connections in adult monkeys with massive sensory loss. *Proc Natl Acad Sci U S A.* 2000 May 9;97(10):5546-50.

Jenkins WM, Merzenich MM, Ochs MT, Allard T, Guic-Robles E. Functional reorganization of primary somatosensory cortex in adult owl monkeys after behaviorally controlled tactile stimulation. *J Neurophysiol* 1990 Jan; 63: 82-104.

Jensen TS, Krebs B, Nielson J, Rasmussen P. Immediate and long-term phantom limb pain in amputees: clinical characteristics and relationship to pre-amputation limb pain. *Pain* 1985 Mar; 21: 407-414

Jones EG. Cortical and subcortical contributions to activity-dependent plasticity in primate somatosensory cortex. *Annu Rev Neurosci* 2000 Apr; 23: 1-37.

Juottonen K, Gockel M, Silen T, Hurri H, Hari R, Forss N. Altered central sensorimotor processing in patients with complex regional pain syndrome. *Pain.* 2002 Aug;98(3):315-23.

Kaas JH. The reorganization of somatosensory and motor cortex after peripheral nerve or spinal cord injury in primates. *Prog Brain Res* 2000; 128: 173-9.

Karl A, Birbaumer N, Lutzenberger W, Cohen LG, Flor H. Reorganization of motor and somatosensory cortex in upper extremity amputees with phantom limb pain. *The Journal of Neuroscience* 2001 May 15, 21 (10): 3069-3618.

Katz J. Psychophysical correlates of phantom limb experience. *J Neurol Neurosurg Psychiatry* 1992 Sep; 55:811-21.

Kenshalo DR Jr, Leonard RB, Chung JM, Willis WD. Facilitation of the responses of primate spinothalmic cells to cold and mechanical stimuli by noxious heating of the skin. *Pain* 1982 Feb ; 12: 141-152.

Kenshalo DR Jr, Leonard RB, Chung JM, Willis WD. Responses of primate spinothalmic neurons to graded and to repeated noxious heat stimuli. *J Neurophysiol* 1979 Sep; 42: 1370-1389.

Kew JJ, Ridding MC, Rothwell RE et al. Reorganization of cortical blood flow and transcranial magnetic stimulation maps in human subjects after upper limb amputation. *J Neorophysiol* 1994 Nov; 71: 2517-24

Kew JJ, Halligan PW, Marshall JC, Passingham RE, Rothwell JC, Ridding MC, et al. Abnormal access of axial vibrotactile input to deafferented somatosensory cortex in human upper limb amputees. *J Neurophysiol* 1997 May; 77: 2753-64.

Knecht S, Soros P, Gurtler S, Imai T, Ringelstein EB, Henningsen H. Phantom sensations following acute pain. *Pain.* 1998 Aug;77(2):209-13.

Knecht S, Henningsen H, Hohling C, Elbert T, Flor H, Pantev C, Taub E. Plasticity of plasticity? Changes in the pattern of perceptual correlates of reorganization after amputation. *Brain.* 1998 Apr;121 (Pt 4):717-24.

Kooijman CM, Dijkstra PU, Geertzen JH, Elzinga A, van der Schans CP. Phantom pain and phantom sensations in upper limb amputees: an epidemiological study. *Pain.* 2000 Jul;87(1):33-41.

Lamour Y, Guilbaud G, Willer JC. Altered properties and laminar distribution of neuronal responses to peripheral stimulation in the Sm 1 Cortex of the arhritic rat. *Brain Res* 1983 Aug; 273: 183-187.

Langlet C, Canu M-H, Falempin M. Short-term reorganization of the rat somatosensory cortex following hypodynamia-hypokinesia. *Neurosc Lett* 1999 May; 266: 145-148.

Lotze M, Laubis-Herrmann U, Topka H, Erb M, Grodd W. Reorganization in the primary motor cortex after spinal cord injury – A functional Magnetic Resonance (fMRI) study. *Restor Neurol Neurosci.* 1999;14(2-3):183-187.

Lotze M, Flor H, Grodd W, Larbig W, Birbaumer N. Phantom movements and pain. An fMRI study in upper limb amputees. *Brain* 2001 Nov; 124: 2268-77

Mauguiere F. [Cervical somatosensory evoked potentials in the healthy subject: analysis of the effect of the location of the reference electrode on aspects of the responses] *Rev Electroencephalogr Neurophysiol Clin.* 1983 Dec;13(3):259-72.

Merzenich MM, Kaas JH, Wall JY, Nelson RJ, Sur M, Felleman DJ. Topographic reorganisation of somatosensory cortical Areas 3b and 1 in adult monkeys following restricted deafferentation. *Neuroscience* 1983 Jan; 8: 33-55.

Merzenich MM, Kaas JH, Wall JY, Sur M, Nelson RJ, Felleman DJ. Progression of change following median nerve section in the cortical representation of the hand in areas 3b and 1 in adult owl and squirrel monkeys. *Neuroscience* 1983 Nov;10: 639-665.

Montoya P, Ritter K, Huse E, Larbig W, Braun C, Topfner S, Lutzenberger W, Grodd W, Flor H, Birbaumer N. The cortical somatotopic map and phantom phenomena in subjects with congenital limb atrophy and traumatic amputees with phantom limb pain. *Eur J Neurosci.* 1998 Mar;10(3):1095-102.

Nicolelis MA, Lin RC, Woodward DJ, Chapin JK. Induction of immediate spatiotemporal changes in thalamic networks by peripheral block of ascending cutaneous information. *Nature.* 1993 Feb 11;361(6412):533-6.

Olausson H, Marchand S, Bittar RG, Bernier J, Ptito A, Bushnell MC. Central pain in a hemispherectomized patient. *Eur J Pain.* 2001;5(2):209-17.

Olausson H, Ha B, Duncan GH, Morin C, Ptito A, Ptito M, Marchand S, Bushnell MC. Cortical activation by tactile and painful stimuli in hemispherectomized patients. *Brain.* 2001 May;124(Pt 5):916-27.

Pascual-Leone A, Torres F. Plasticity of sensorimotor cortex representation of the reading finger in Braille readers. *Brain* 1993 Feb; 116: 39-52.

Pascual-Leone A, Cohen LG, Brasil-Neto JP, Hallett M. Non-invasive differentiation of motor cortical representation of hand muscles by mapping of optimal current directions. *Electroencephalogr Clin Neurophysiol* 1994 Feb; 93: 42-8.

Pascual-Leone A, Dang N, Cohen LG, Brasil-Neto JP, Cammarota A, Hallett M. Modulation of muscle responses evoked by transcranial magnetic stimulation during the acquisition of new fine motor skills. *J Neurophysiol 1995* Sep; 74: 1037-1045.

Pascual-Leone A, Wassermann EM, Sadato N, Hallett M. The role of reading activity on the modulation of motor cortical outputs to the reading hand in Braille readers. *Ann Neurol* 1995 Dec; 38: 910-915.

Pascual-Leone A, Peris M, Tormos JM, Pascual AP, Catala MD. Reorganization of human cortical motor output maps following traumatic forearm amputation. *Neuroreport* 1996 Sep; 7: 2068-70.

Pascual-Leone A, Tormos JM, Keenan J, Tarazona F, Canete C, Catala MD. Study and modulation of human cortical excitability with transcranial magnetic stimulation. *J Clin Neurophysiol.* 1998 Jul;15(4):333-43.

Perl ER, Kumuzawa T, Lynn B, Kenins P. Sensitization of high threshod receptors with unmyelinated (C) afferent fibres. *Progress in Brain Research* 1976; 43: 263-277.

Pettit MJ, Schwark HD. Receptive field organisation in dorsal column nuclei during temporary denervation. *Science 1*993 Dec; 262: 2054-2056.

Peyron R, Laurent B, García-Larrea L. Functional imaging of brain responses to pain. A review and meta-analysis. *Neurophysiol Clin* 2000 Oct; 30: 263-88

Pons T, Garraghty PE, Ommaya AK, Kaas JH, Taub E, Mishkin M. Massive cortical reorganization after sensory deafferentation in adult macaques. *Science* 1991 Jun 28; 252: 1857-1860.

Price DD, Hayes RL, Ruda M, Dubner R. Spatial and temporal transformations of input to spinothalamic tract neurons and their relation to somatic sensations. *J Neurophysiol* 1978 Jul; 41: 933-946.

Raisman G, Field PM. A quantitative investigation of the developement of collateral reinnervation after partial deafferentation of the septal nuclei. *Proc Natl Acad Sci USA* 1988; 85: 2003-7.

Ramachandran VS, Stewart M, Rogers-Ramachandran DC. Perceptual correlates of massive cortical reorganization. *Neuroreport.* 1992 Jul;3(7):583-6.

Recanzone GH, Jenkins WM, Hradek GT, Merzenich MM. Progressive improvement in discriminative abilities in adult owl monkeys performing a tactile frequency discrimination task. *J Neurophysiol* 1992 May 67: 1015-1030.

Recanzone GH, Merzenich MM, Jenkins WM. Frequency discrimination training engaging a restricted skin surface results in emergence of a cutaneous response zone in cortical area 3a. *J Neurophysio*l 1992 May ; 67: 1057-1070.

Recanzone GH, Merzenich MM, Jenkins WM, Grajski KA, Dinse HR. Topographic reorganisation of the hand representation in cortical area 3b in owl monkeys trained in a frequency-discrimination task. *J Neurophysiol* 1992 May 67: 1031-1056.

Recanzone GH, Merzenich MM, Schreiner CE. Changes in the distributed temporal response properties of S1 cortical neurons reflect improvements in performance on a temporally based tactile discrimination task. *J Neurophysiol* 1992 May ; 67: 1071-1091.

Rossini PM, Martino G, Narici L, Pasquarelli A, Peresson M, Pizzella V, et al. Short-term brain plasticity in humans: transient finger representation changes in sensory cortex somatotopy following ischemic anaesthesia. *Brain Res* 1994Apr; 642: 169-177.

Rossini PM, Rossi S, Tecchio F, Pasqualetti P, Finazzi-Agrò A, Sabato A. Focal brain stimulation in healthy humans: motor maps changes following partial hand sensory deprivation. *Neurosci Lett* 1996 Aug; 214: 191-195.

Rosso T, Aglioti SM, Zanette G, Ischia S, Finco G, Farina S, Fiaschi A, Tinazzi M. Functional plasticity in the human primary somatosensory cortex following acute lesion of the anterior lateral spinal cord: neurophysiological evidence of short-term cross-modal plasticity. *Pain.* 2003 Jan;101(1-2):117-27.

Rothwell JC, Thompson PD, Day BL, Boyd S, Marsden CD. Stimulation of the human motor cortex through the scalp. *Exp Physiol.* 1991 Mar;76(2):159-200.

Sadato N, Zeffiro TA, Campbell G, Konishi J, Shibasaki H, Hallett M. Regional cerebral blood flow changes in motor cortical areas after transient anesthesia of the forearm. *Ann Neurol.* 1995 Jan;37(1):74-81.

Schroeder CE, Seto S, Arezzo JC, Garraghty PE. Electrophysiological evidence for overlapping dominant and latent inputs to somatosensory cortex in squirrel monkeys. *J Neurophysiol.* 1995 Aug;74(2):722-32.

Schroeder CE, Steinschneider M, Javitt DC, Tenke CE, Givre SJ, Mehta AD, Simpson GV, Arezzo JC, Vaughan HG Jr. Localization of ERP generators and identification of underlying neural processes. *Electroencephalogr Clin Neurophysiol Suppl.* 1995;44:55-75.

Sherman RA, Sherman CJ. Prevalence and characteristics of chronic phantom limb pain among American veterans. Results of a trial survey. *Am J Phys Med.* 1983 Oct;62(5):227-38.

Sherman RA, Sherman CJ, Parker L. Chronic phantom and stump pain among American veterans: results of a survey. *Pain.* 1984 Jan;18(1):83-95

Sherman RA. Stump and phantom limb pain. *Neurol Clin.* 1989 May;7(2):249-64.

Simone DA, Sorkin LS, Oh U, Chung JM, Owens C, La Motte RH, Willis WD. Neurogenic hyperalgesia: central correlates in responses of spinothalamic tract neurons. *J Neurophysiol* 1991 Jul ;66: 228-246.

Sörös P, Knecht S, Bantel C, Imai T, Wüsten R, Pantev C, Lütkenhöner B, Bükle H, Henningsen H. Functional reorganization of the human primary somatosensory cortex after acute pain demonstred by magnetoencephalography. *Neurosci Lett* 2001 Feb; 298: 195-8.

Svensson P, Rosenberg B, Beydoun A, Morrow TJ, Casey KL. Comparative psychophysical characteristics of cutaneous CO2 laser and contact heat stimulation. *Somatosens Mot Res.* 1997;14(2):113-8.

Svensson P, Beydoun A, Morrow TJ, Casey KL. Non-painful and painful stimulation of human skin and muscle: analysis of cerebral evoked potentials. *Electroencephalogr Clin Neurophysiol.* 1997 Jul;104(4):343-50.

Svensson P, Minoshima S, Beydoun A, Morrow TJ, Casey KL. Cerebral processing of acute skin and muscle pain in humans. *J Neurophysiol.* 1997 Jul;78(1):450-60.

Talbot JD, Marrett S, Evans AC, Meyer E, Bushnell MC, Duncan GH Multiple representations of pain in human cerebral cortex. *Science.* 1991 Mar 15;251(4999):1355-8.

Tinazzi M, Zanette G, Polo A, Volpato D, Manganotti P, Bonato C, Testoni R, Fiaschi A. Transient deafferentation in humans induces rapid modulation of primary sensory cortex not associated with subcortical changes: a somatosensory evoked potential study. *Neurosci Lett* 1997 Feb; 223: 21-24.

Tinazzi M, Zanette G, Volpato D, Testoni R, Bonato C, Manganotti P, Miniussi C, Fiaschi A. Neurophysiological evidence of neuroplasticity at multiple levels of the somatosensory system in patients with carpal tunnel syndrome. *Brain* 1998 Sep; 121: 1785-1794.

Tinazzi M, Fiaschi A, Rosso T, Faccioli F, Grosslercher J, Aglioti SM. Neuroplastic changes related to pain occur at multiple levels of the human somatosensory system: A somatosensory-evoked potentials study in patients with cervical radicular pain.*J Neurosci.* 2000 Dec 5;20(24):9277-83.

Tinazzi M, Rosso T, Zanette G, Fiaschi A, Aglioti SM. Rapid modulation of cortical proprioceptive activity induced by transient cutaneous deafferentation: neurophysiological evidence of short-term plasticity. across different somatosensory modalities in humans. *Eur J Neurosci.* 2003 Dec;18(11):3053-60.

Tinazzi M, Valeriani M, Moretto G, Rosso T, Nicolato A, Fiaschi A, Aglioti SM. Plastic interactions between hand and face cortical representations in patients with trigeminal neuralgia: a somatosensory-evoked potentials study. *Neuroscience.* 2004;127(3):769-76.

Valeriani M, Arendt-Nielsen L, Le Pera D, Restuccia D, Rosso T, De Armas L, Maiese T, Fiaschi A, Tonali P, Tinazzi M. Short-term plastic changes of the human nociceptive system following acute pain induced by capsaicin. *Clinical Neurophys* 2003 Oct; 114: 1879-90.

Valeriani M, Tinazzi M, Le Pera D, Restuccia D, De Armas L, Maiese T, Tonali P, Arendt-Nielsen L. Inhibitory effect of capsaicin evoked trigeminal pain on warmth sensation and warmth evoked potentials. *Exp Brain Res.* 2005 Jan; 160 (1): 29-37.

Wall PD, Egger MD. Formation of new connexions in adult rat brains after partial deafferentation. *Nature.* 1971 Aug 20;232(5312):542-5.

Wang X, Merzenich MM, Sameshima K, Jenkins WM. Remodelling of hand representation in adult cortex determined by timing of tactile stimulation. *Nature* 1995; 378: 71-74.

Wartan SW, Hamann W, Wedley JR, McColl I. Phantom pain and sensation among British veteran amputees.*Br J Anaesth.* 1997 Jun;78(6):652-9.

Willoch F, Rosen G, Tolle TR, Oye I, Wester HJ, Berner N, Schwaiger M, Bartenstein P. Phantom limb pain in the human brain: unraveling neural circuitries of phantom limb sensations using positron emission tomography. *Ann Neurol.* 2000 Dec;48(6):842-9.

Xerri C, Merzenich MM, Jenkins W, Santucci S. Representational plasticity in cortical area 3b paralleling tactual-motor skill acquisition in adult monkeys. *Cereb Cortex* 1999 Apr-May; 9: 264-76.

Yang TT, Gallen CC, Ramachandran J, Cobb S, Schwartz BJ, Bloom FE. Non-invasive detection of cerebral plasticity in adult human somatosensory cortex. *Neuroreport* 1994 Feb; 5: 701-704.

Zanette G, Tinazzi M, Manganotti P, Bonato C, Polo A. Two distinct cervical N13 potentials are evoked by ulnar nerve stimulation. *Electroencephalogr Clin Neurophysiol.* 1995 Mar;96(2):114-20.

In Frontiers in Pain Research
Editor: Alexendre Lucas, pp.133-156

ISBN 1-59454-828-5

Chapter 7

THE AFFECTIVE AND COGNITIVE DIMENSION OF NOCICEPTION IN AN ANIMAL MODEL: THE ROLE OF THE ANTERIOR CINGULATE CORTEX

Francisco Pellicer,* Edgar Torres-López, Francisco Sotres-Bayón, Alberto López-Avila, Ulises Coffeen, J. Manuel Ortega-Legasp and Rosendo del Ángel

Laboratorio de Neurofisiología Integrativa, Dirección de Neurociencias,
Instituto Nacional de Psiquiatría Ramón de la Fuente, México

ABSTRACT

The relationship between the cingulum and the processing of emotions was first established by Papez in the 1930's. Since then, many studies have related the cingulum bundle to areas of the limbic system that constitute a circuit which includes the hippocampus, the mamillary bodies, the anterior thalamic nucleus and the cingulate cortex. Some studies have associated limbic structures with cognitive and affective pain processing. For more than four decades, the cingulotomy has been used in the treatment of patients with central or intractable pain or who exhibit refractority to pharmacological treatment to pain.

Recent findings including those of functional image studies highlight the activation of limbic structures such as the thalamus, anterior cingulate cortex (ACC), insular cortex and mesolimbic dopaminergic nuclei in central pain processing. This evidence makes relevant the animal experimental study of loci, pathways, neurotransmitters and receptors regarding the relationship between the limbic system and chronic central neuropathic pain.

---

* Correspondence to: Francisco Pellicer, Instituto Nacional de Psiquiatría Ramón de la Fuente, Camino a Xochimilco 101 San Lorenzo Huipulco Tlalpan, C.P. 14370, México, D.F., México. pellicer@imp.edu.mx Tel: +52 55 56553232, Fax: +52 55 56559980

The experiments were performed based on the somatic inflammatory process (hind paw carrageenan injection) and peripheral denervation (thermonociception prior to sciatic transection), both which trigger quantifiable chronic nociception that is expressed either as autotomy behaviour (AB) or self injury behaviour (SIB).
The results have shown that the electrical stimulation of the cingulum bundle simultaneously to an inflammatory painful process accelerates the onset and enhances the rate of autotomy induced by hind paw carrageenan injections. Moreover, an electrical stimulation of the anteriomedial and mediodorsal thalamic nuclei, which is the origin of the cingulum bundle and whose glutamatergic afferents have been widely described, also enhances incidence and shorten onset as well as increase intensity of AB.
The ACC is directly innervated through the medial forebrain bundle by the ventral tegmental area (VTA), which is a dopaminergic nucleus in which pain modulation is involved. As far as another approach is concerned, the role of the VTA and dopamine in the modulation of chronic nociception involved in AB was tested. In this sense, the electrical stimulation of the VTA diminishes AB, whereas its lesion enhances it. The direct microinjection of dopamine into the ACC has the same effect as the VTA stimulation. To sum up, the activation of the glutamatergic afferents to the ACC coming from the anterior thalamus nuclei enhance AB, whereas the activation of dopaminergic ones coming from the VTA diminish it.
Furthermore, experiments regarding the relationship between the specific receptors of the dopaminergic and glutamatergic systems within the ACC in the genesis and maintenance of chronic nociception measured as AB show that an N-methyl-d-aspartate (NMDA) receptor antagonist (MK801) and amantadine (NMDA receptor antagonist and dopamine releaser), both diminish AB.
In this chapter, the memory mechanisms associated with the ACC and related to their consolidation will also be reviewed. In this matter, AB is susceptible of being diminished by a muscarinic blockade of cholinergic transmission using scopolamine.

LIMBIC SYSTEM AND PAIN PERCEPTION

The neuroanatomic and functional relationship in which the limbic system is involved has historically been difficult to define. The relationship between the cingulum and the processing of emotions was first established by Papez in the 1930's (Papez 1937). Nevertheless, Vogt has proposed an emblematic dichotomy in the cingulate gyrus (Devinsky et al. 1995; Vogt et al. 1992). This dichotomy involves structure and function in spite of the fact that the whole structure plays a role in limbic functions. On one hand, the caudal cingulate gyrus is related to visuospatial and memory functions. On the other, there is the rostral part which is of most relevance for our interest due to the fact that it is engaged in executive functions associated with the affective sphere. The rostral limbic system is constituted by structures such as the amygdala and septum, orbitofrontal, anterior insula and anterior cingulate cortices, the ventral striatum including the accumbens nucleus and severeal brainstem motor nuclei such as the periaqueductal grey matter (for review refer to Devinsky, 1995). It is relevant to note that most of those structures play a significant role in the cognitive-affective component of pain (Abbott and Melzack 1978).

There is a neurosurgical finding that was reported over 50 years ago which evidences the cognitive-affective relationship between the anterior cingulate cortex (ACC) and pain perception. Thus, patients who exhibit refractory pain states to pharmacological treatment have been successfully treated with cingulotomy. Such patients report that they continue to feel the pain but it does not bother them or trigger any adverse emotional reaction (Foltz and White 1962). In fact, the perception of pain as such does not appear to be modified but most of the patients state that they continue to have it but it was not particularly bothersome, "doesn't worry me".

The Pain Image in the Brain

Jones and Derbyshire (1993) have discussed in a previous report that there are indeed significant and consistent changes in regional cerebral blood flow in response to experimental acute nociception. The involved structures are the thalamus and lentiform nucleus, anterior cingulate, prefrontal and insular cortices.

Morphine has been proposed to predominantely reduce the affective components of pain without altering its somatosensory localization. Nevertheless, morphine is widely understood as a pain killer, which would imply that patients under its effects express no pain sensation. This was tested by measuring regional cerebral blood flow and the results showed that the anterior cingulate and prefrontal and insular cortices had a reduced flow whereas there were no changes in the somatosensory cortex (Jones and Derbyshire 1993).

Experimental protocols regarding pain are normally carried out first in animal models. In an inverse fashion, the first experimental functional image studies (functional magnetic resonance, positron emission tomography, single photon emission computed tomography) were performed in humans due to the fact that the first available technology was suitable only for human beings. Later on, the appropriate functional image technology capable of reproducing high resolution and teslage functional images in animals was developed. These techniques applied in animal experimental approaches show that the ACC is activated by nociceptive electrical or chemical stimuli in an analogous way to humans. (Chang and Shyu 2001; Tuor et al. 2000). This fact implies that less evolved species, such as the rat, activate the same functional condition (locus and physiological mechanisms) for the affective and cognitive dimension of pain.

Considering the previous evidence regarding the activation of the above mentioned central structures in long lasting nociception processing it is relevant to review the neurophysiological mechanisms involved in such activation.

Experimental Models in Chronic Nociception

Experimental research in chronic nociception using whole animals is an approach plagued with methodological drawbacks within the ethical realm, as well as difficulties in the analysis and interpretation of time dependent results (Albe-Fessard et al. 1990; Levitt 1985; Zeltser and Seltzer 1994). In relation to this matter, we believe that an experimental model for the study of chronic nociception must comply with the following criteria: (a) The experimental model must be reasonably similar to the human phenomenon. (b) The model should provide the intrinsic mechanisms to gain some insight in the phenomenon under study.

(c) The experiments must fulfil the norms and ethical standard criteria established for pain research (Zimmerman 1983). In this sense, numerous models of peripheral neuropathy have been created in rat that achieve this aim either by neurocompression at different nerve levels (Bennett and Xie 1988; Kim and Chung 1992; Seltzer et al. 1990) or denervation (Wall et al. 1979). These models produce chronic nociception manifested as autotomy behaviour (AB) towards the limb associated to the neuropathy. In the model devised by Wall et al (1979) daily autotomy scores are computed, giving a score of 1 for the removal of one or more nails; an additional score of 1 for each distal half digit attacked and a further score of 1 for each proximal half digit attacked. If the distal or proximal half of the paw are attacked an additional score of 1 is added for each one. These procedures have made the study of the putative role of brain structures possible (Vaccarino and Melzack 1991), as well as that of peripheral and central mechanisms of the nervous system involved in the development of chronic nociception.

In this sense, our group has developed an experimental model that displays a quantifiable self-injury behaviour (SIB) produced by the inflammation of soft tissue located in the paw of the rat elicited by carrageenan infiltration and presents an *ad integrum* behavioural recovery response (López-Avila et al. 2004b; Pellicer et al. 1999; Sotres-Bayón et al. 2001; Torres-López et al. 2000).

Considering the above mentioned experimental frameworks as useful tools for the research on chronic pain, several experimental approaches were developed in order to answer the role, connections, neurotransmitters and receptors within the anterior cingulate cortex involved in long lasting central nociception measured as autotomy (AB) or self injury (SIB) behaviours.

All the experiments reported in this chapter that were performed by our group were conducted in agreement with the ethics committee regulations of the International Association for the Study of Pain (Zimmerman 1983) and with the bioethical commission of the Instituto Nacional de Psiquiatría Ramón de la Fuente (INPRF).

The Role of the ACC in Chronic Nociception: Experimental Approaches

Among the central starting points that were considered to answer long lasting central nociception it is relevant to mention a work that reports that the infiltration of local anaesthetics in the boundary of the cingulum in rats previously neurectomised, interrupts the information pathways through this bundle, producing a disruption in the initiation and subsequent maintenance of the neural processes related to autotomy which occurrence was significantly reduced and also the intensity diminished and onset delayed (Magnusson and Vaccarino 1996; Vaccarino and Melzack 1991).

In this context we decided to perform electrical stimulation in the cingulum bundle under the rationale of potentiating self injury behaviour. The experimental design permitted us to distinguish whether SIB was produced by either the electrical stimulation on its own, with the induction of an inflammatory process using carrageenan two days after the last stimulation or with the stimulation and the inflammatory process simultaneously. Electrical stimulation *per se* did not induce autotomy. Nevertheless, after the induction of the inflammatory process, different degrees of autotomy were presented. The highest autotomy score can be achieved by stimulating at the same time of the induction of the inflammatory process. This experimental findings have lead to the conclusion that the triggering factor of SIB is the presence of a specific painful somatosensorial reference (inflammatory painful process) defined by our group as sensorial quality. This sensorial quality is a fundamental condition for the beginning of SIB (Pellicer et al. 1999) (Figures 1 and 2).

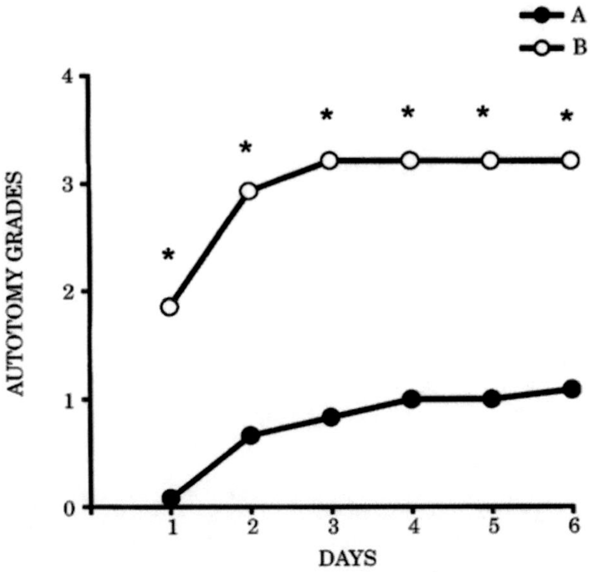

Figure 1. The graph shows the temporal course of autotomy. The sham group (filled circles n = 12) was implanted with electrodes but not stimulated, with hind paw carrageenan induced inflammation. The experimental group (open circles n = 14) had the cingulum bundle electrically stimulated 10 minutes daily for 5 days and the carrageenan injection and first stimulation were performed simultaneously. The ordinates represents the lesions caused by autotomy in grades: grade 1, single lesion of the major longitudinal axis less than 3 mm; grade 2, multiple lesions of the major longitudinal axis less than 3 mm; grade 3, single lesion of the major longitudinal axis larger than 3mm; grade 4, multiple lesions of the major longitudinal axis larger than 3 mm. The abscissa is the time. Notice the highest value of autotomy is shown by the electrical stimulated group. The data reveals a statistical significant difference between these two groups, Student-Newman-Keuls Least Significant Rank test. F-value =2.683 $^*P < 0.05$.

Another important fact is to establish the nuclei and neuroanatomical connections that regard the cingulum bundle and nociceptive sensations.

The ACC receives projections from the anteriomedial (AM) (Domesick 1972; Horikawa et al. 1988; Shibata and Kato 1993) and lateral mediodorsal (MD) nuclei (Groenewegen 1988; Krettek and Price 1977) of the thalamus through the cingulum bundle and the anterior limb of the internal capsule (Domesick 1970). Electrophysiological studies have provided evidence for the existence of nociceptive neurons in the ACC (Mantz et al. 1988; Sikes and Vogt 1992; Vogt et al. 1992; Yamamura et al. 1996) that respond in an excitatory fashion to the electrical stimulation of the MD nucleus (Dostrovsky and Guilbaud 1990; Hsu and Shyu 1997; Mantz et al. 1988). Also, neurons of the AM and MD nuclei receive nociceptive input (Rinaldi et al.

1991). There is evidence that excitatory aminoacids are involved as neurotransmitters in these pathways (Gigg et al. 1992; Pirot et al. 1994). In this sense, the electrical simulation of the MD and AM nuclei has proven to modify nociceptive information processing. Thus, AM and MD stimulated animals show an enhanced incidence and shortened onset as well as increased intensity of SIB. This fact proves that the electrical stimulation of the AM nucleus, in the presence of the sensorial quality, produces the highest SIB score as compared to intralaminar, reticular and stria medularis stimulation (Figure 3A). MD stimulation also produces an important SIB score, although less evident than the one obtained by AM stimulation (Figure 3B). These results showed for the first time that the AM and MD nuclei play a relevant role in the cognitive-affective component of pain (Torres-López et al. 2000).

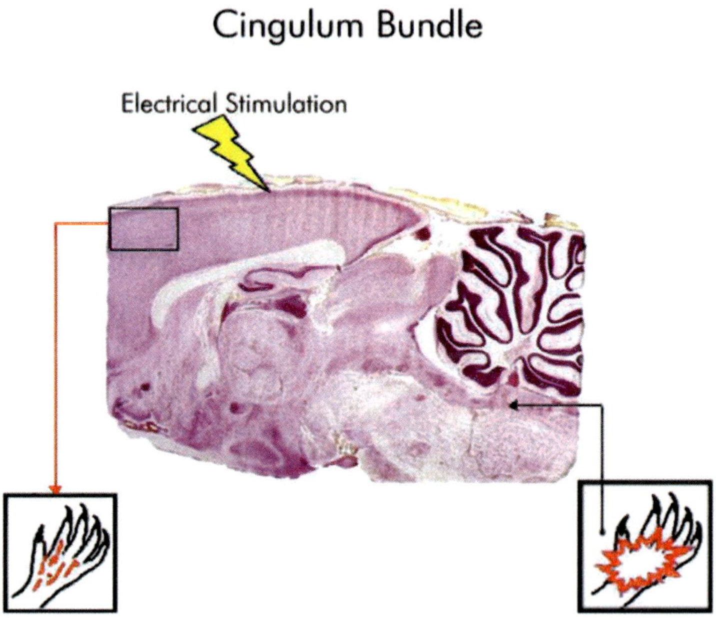

Figure 2. The electrical stimulation of the cingulum bundle increases self injury behaviour triggered by an inflammatory process induced by the infiltration of carrageenan in the hind paw. Stimulation parameters: square pulses of 0.2 ms at 100 Hz for 1 s every 5 s; the current was adjusted for each animal, with an average of 110 uA.

Another important system which projects monosynapically from the ventral tegmental area (VTA) via the anterior-medial forebrain bundle into the ACC is the mesolimbic dopaminergic system. The VTA is one of the nuclei that are now considered to be part of the basal ganglia (BG), which have been traditionally related to the control of motor responses but nevertheless are considered as being involved in the processing of noxious somatosensorial information. There are evidences indicating that the VTA is an important nucleus for pain modulation. This structure participates in various neural circuits that are involved in induced analgesia by electrical stimulation (Mayer and Liebeskind 1974; Mayer and Price 1976), stress (Thierry et al. 1976), morphine (Morgan and Franklin 1990) and also electroacupuncture (Ma et al. 1993). Moreover, it has been suggested that the VTA participates in what sometimes is called dissociative analgesia (Franklin 1989), in which the affective component of pain is lost.

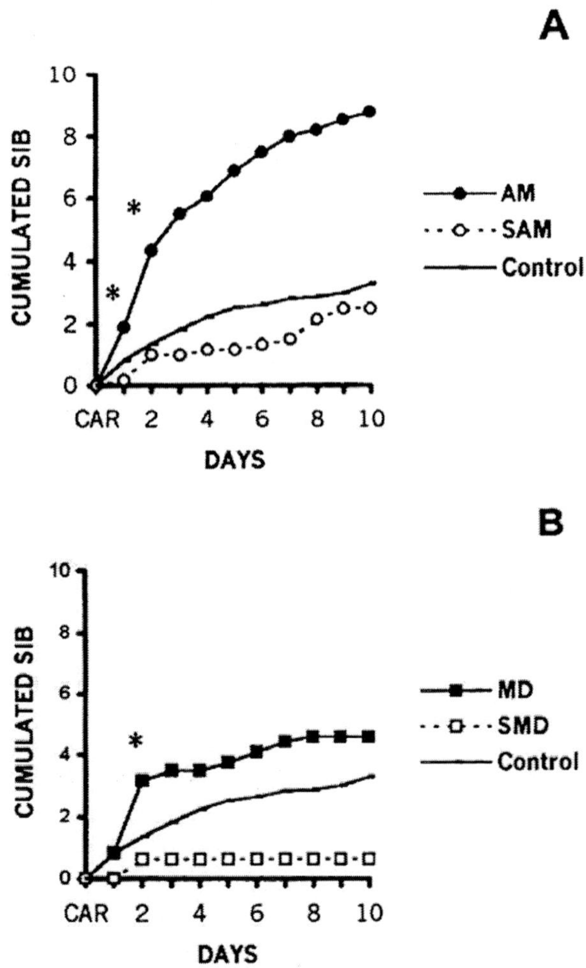

Figure 3. Evolution of the cumulative SIB. (A) AM (n = 17), AM sham (n = 8 SAM, microelectrode implanted but not electrically stimulated), and control (microelectrode not implanted) groups. The AM group had the greatest self-injury activity (shows the highest slope in the curve) in the first 2 days after carrageenan injection. (B) MD (n = 12), MD sham (n = 7, SMD) and control groups (n = 17). The MD group had greater self-injury activity than the SMD and control groups in the second day after the carrageenan injection. Student-Newman-Keuls Significant Range * $p<0.05$. For stimulation parameters refer to Figure 2.

In experiments that evaluate persistent pain by means of pain related behaviours in the rat, contradictory results have been reported for the effects of electrical stimulation and lesion of the VTA. It has been shown that a neurochemical lesion of the VTA produced by the injection of 6-hydroxy-dopamine, increases the behavioural response to pain, triggered by denervation (Saade et al. 1997) and reduces the behavioural response to the formalin test (Morgan and Franklin 1990). On the other hand, contradictory results have been reported for electrical stimulation of the VTA. Thus, Gorea and Lombard (Gorea and Lombard 1984) reported an increase in autotomy behaviour, while Sarkis et al. (Sarkis et al. 1984) showed that autotomy diminishes after VTA self stimulation.

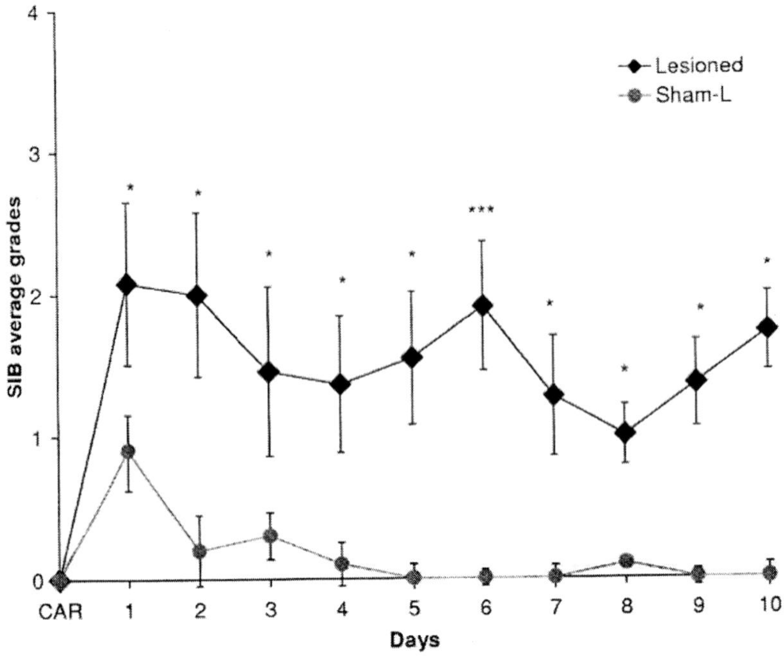

Figure 4. Effect of ventral tegmental area (VTA) radiofrequency lesion on self injury behaviour (SIB). An increase in the average of the SIB grades in the lesioned group (n = 10) as compared to the Sham-L group (n = 10) was observed through 10 days of the behavioural evaluation (MANOVA, F=21.493, α=0.000). Student's *t*-test (*P<=0.05; *** P<=0.000). the values represent SIB mean grades (±S.D.). Sham-L, sham of the lesion experiment.

Considering the importance of the VTA as a pain modulator in what has been suggested to be the neural substrate of dissociative and induced analgesia, and given the established controversies of the aforementioned results, another experiment was performed in which this nucleus was lesioned using radiofrequency and was electrically stimulated before or after the induction of a nociceptive stimlulus (carrageenan infiltrated into the right hind paw) to see its distinctive analgesic effect on a persistent pain related behavioural response in which SIB was measured (Sotres-Bayón et al. 2001).

The results of this study show that VTA experimental manipulations (radiofrequency lesion or stimulation after the application of the nociceptive stimulus) modify the SIB. The suppression of VTA output by its lesion enhances the occurrence of SIB, a pain related behaviour (Figures 4 and 5); while the activation of the same nucleus by electrical stimulation after the induction of the nociceptive stimulus, but not before, facilitates analgesic processes, expressed as a diminished SIB (Figure 5). Thus, these results suggest that the VTA is an important brain structure involved in the processing and modulation of persistent pain information.

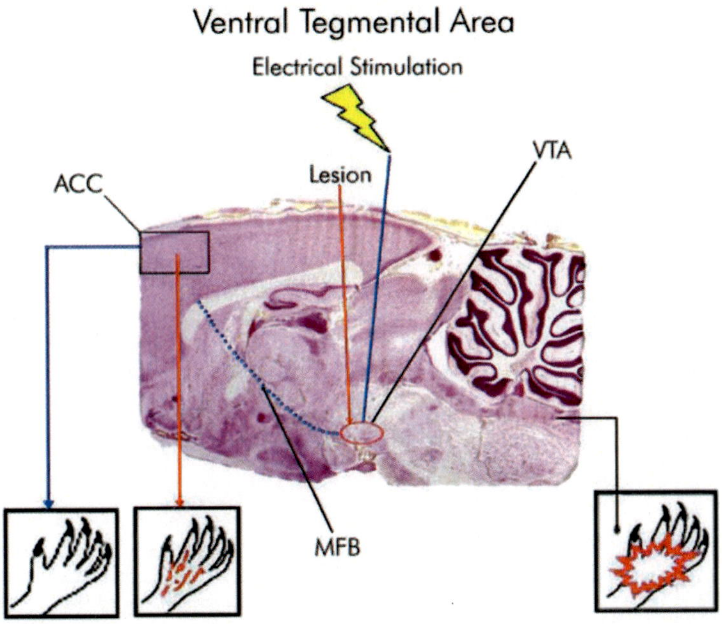

Figure 5. The ventral tegmental area (VTA) reaches the anterior cingulate cortex (ACC) through the medial forebrain bundle (MFB). The bilateral radiofrequency lesion of the VTA (A10) increases self injury behaviour triggered by an inflammatory process induced by the infiltration of carrageenan in the hind paw. On the other hand, its electrical stimulation diminishes it. For stimulation parameters refer to Figure 2.

In this context, it was relevant to investigate the role that dopaminergic and glutamatergic systems might play within the ACC in the onset and evolution of chronic nociception. With this framework, the use of microinjected dopamine, and an N-methyl-d-aspartate (NMDA) receptor antagonist into the ACC was decided. Due to the pharmacological properties of these two systems amantadine was also used. This drug is a low affinity non competitive NMDA receptor antagonist with fast block and unblock kinetics (Kornhuber et al. 1991; Kornhuber et al. 1995). Besides, there is evidence of the role of amantadine as a dopaminergic releaser (Gordon et al. 1996; Stone 1976; Takahashi et al. 1996; Toide 1990). As in previous experimental series, these experiments were performed by a sciatic neurectomy employed as a trigger for neuropathic pain expressed as autotomy behaviour (AB) in the rat (Wall et al. 1979). The nociceptive process was increased by a painful stimulation (thermonociception) applied prior to denervation in order to enhance the AB (Coderre and Melzack 1986; López-Avila et al. 1999). The results regarding this experiment are discussed as follows:

Dopamine and the ACC

The findings suggest that dopaminergic mesocortical circuits within the ACC are able to inhibit long-term nociception related to mesocortical pathways (Figure 6). Such a role is not limited to the ACC since dopamine is an important inhibitor of nociception throughout the cerebral cortex (Burkey et al. 1999). As far as the dopamine dose is concerned, the microinjections of nanomolar doses of dopamine were the most effective in diminishing the autotomy score, whereas micro and millimolar doses were less effective. This is in agreement with previous evidence showing that dopamine release within the ACC and the striatum induced by chemical noxious stimulation of the rat's hind paw, or stress induced by an electrical tail shock is in the order of pico to nanomoles (Abercrombie et al. 1989; Gao et al. 2001). However, the results show an inverse dose dependent effect. The micro and millimolar doses are less effective in antinociception than the nanomolar concentration. Based on the data obtained in the discussed work, the lack of effect on autotomy score when using higher doses of dopamine is unable of being supported. Nevertheless, it seems possible that, as reported by Fuster, the lack of pre-synaptic dopamine receptors in the mesolimbic system prevents a regulation of dopamine action through this mechanism (Fuster 1997). Moreover, since extracellular dopamine increase can reduce post-synaptic receptor expression (Morelli et al. 1993), the subsequent desensitization would be sufficient to reduce the effect of dopamine on ACC neurons.

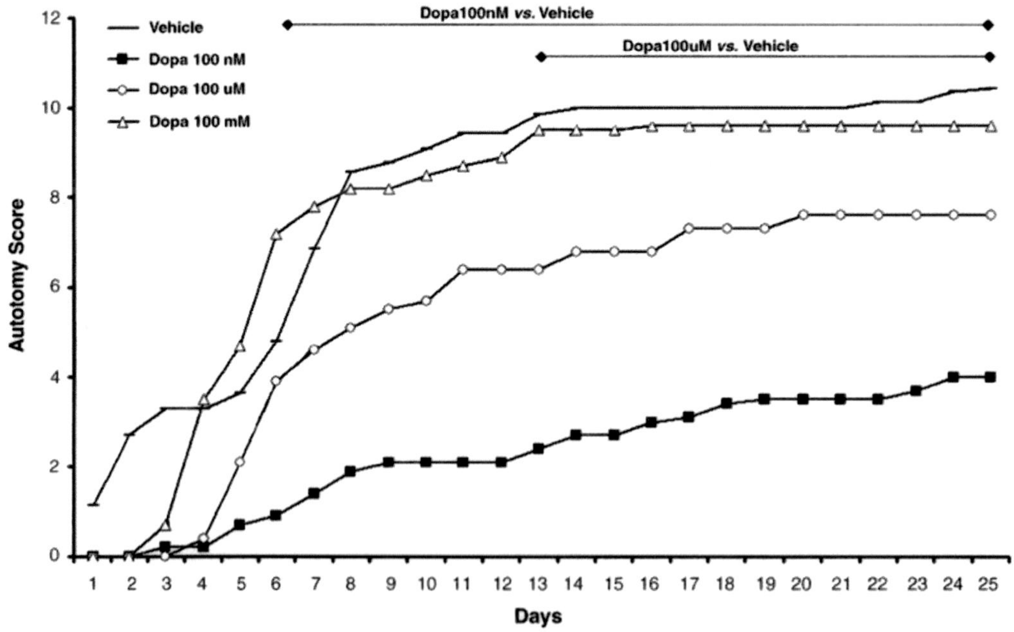

Figure 6. Long-term nociceptive response measured through autotomy score for 25 days. Vehicle group (n=14) with the induction of a nociceptive process (rat's right hind paw immersed in water at 55 °C for 20 s), denervation 30 min afterwards and 2 ul saline solution microinjection into the ACC after denervation. Dopa (n = 10 each) with the microinjection of 2 ul of dopamine 100 nM, 100 uM and 100 mM, respectively. A significant decrease in autotomy score in groups dopa 100 nM and 100 uM is observed when compared to the vehicle group (repeated measures Anova $p < 0.05$). The significance between groups per day was established by a Tukey test as a post hoc ($p < 0.05$) (horizontal bars).

NMDA RECEPTOR AND THE ACC

Antinociceptive effects of NMDA receptor antagonists in the central nervous system (CNS) have been shown following several routes of administration (Carpenter and Dickenson 1999; Dickenson 1997; Eide 2000a; Eide 2000b; Lutfy et al. 1997; Nikolajsen et al. 1996). Our results showed a significant decrease in nociception following the microinjection of an NMDA receptor antagonist (MK801) within the ACC at both nanomolar and millimolar concentrations (López-Avila et al. 2004a) (Figure 7). Such doses have been shown to elicit antinociceptive effects in other CNS areas (Luger et al. 1995; Nasstrom et al. 1993). These results suggest the participation of NMDA receptors in the ACC in the genesis of long-term nociception mediated through AB.

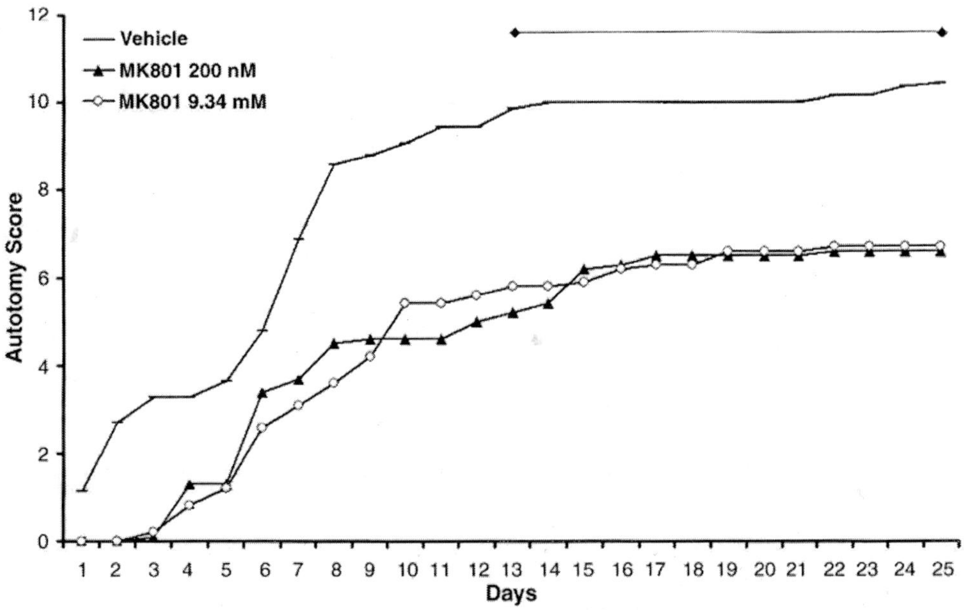

Figure 7. Long-term nociceptive response measured through autotomy score for 25 days. Vehicle (n= 14). Groups MK 801, microinjected with 2 ul of MK 801 200 nM (n = 9) and 9.34 mM (n = 10). A significant decrease in autotomy score in both MK 801 groups is observed when compared to vehicle (repeated measures Anova $p < 0.05$). The difference between MK801 groups vs. vehicle per day was established by a Tukey test as a post hoc ($p < 0.05$) (horizontal bar).

AMANTADINE AND THE ACC

The findings show that a single microinjection of amantadine into the ACC reduces significantly long-term nociception measured as AB (Figure 8). Amantadine was microinjected at two different times in order to investigate whether it has a prophylactic, therapeutic or both actions. The results suggest a similar prophylactic and therapeutic effect of amantadine within a time lapse of 30 min prior to denervation to immediately after it.

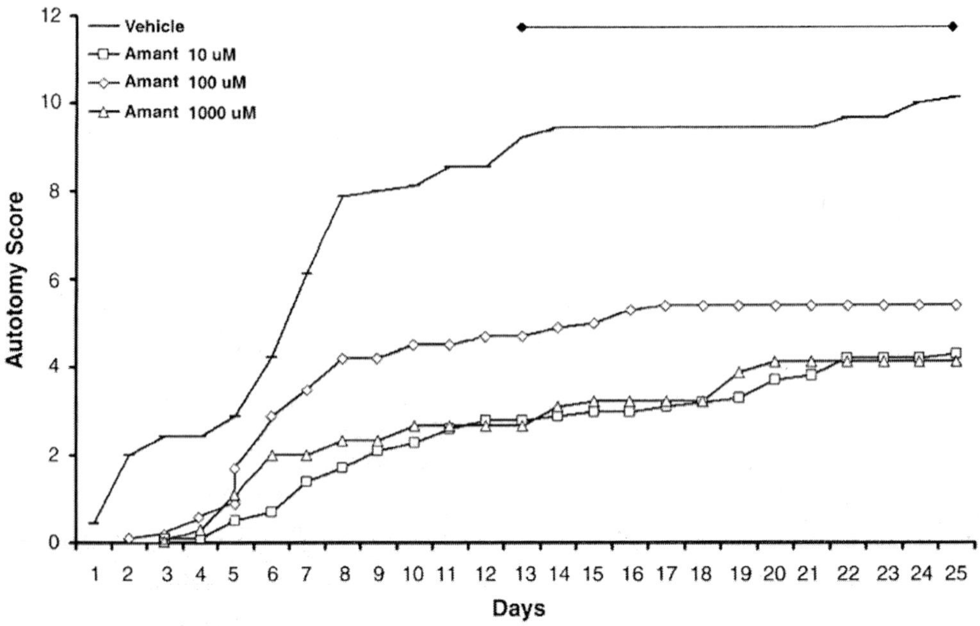

Figure 8. Long-term nociceptive response measured through autotomy score for 25 days. Vehicle (n = 14). Groups amant, microinjected with 2 ul of amantadine 10 (n = 10), 100 (n = 10) and 1000 uM (n = 9), 30 min prior to denervation. A significant decrease in autotomy score in all amantadine groups is observed when compared vehicle (repeated measures ANOVA $p < 0.05$). The difference between the amantadine groups vs. vehicle per day was established by a Tukey test as a post hoc ($p < 0.05$) (horizontal bar).

Despite not being a significant difference between groups, the experiments in which amantadine was administered prior to denervation showed a lower autotomy score than its post-denervation counterparts. The antinociceptive effects of amantadine into the ACC could be related to its dual pharmacological properties. The first one relates to its capability of blocking NMDA receptors. A number of studies have shown that NMDA receptor blockade diminishes central sensitization (Eide 2000a; Eide 2000b). Moreover, the administration of NMDA antagonists prior or during the induction of a nociceptive process, as seen in the above discussed experiment (Figure 7), is able to reduce nociception (Bennett 1994; Davar et al. 1991; Dickenson 1997; Eisenberg et al. 1994; Herrero et al. 1994; Khandwala et al. 1997; Kristensen et al. 1992; Lutfy et al. 1997; Mao et al. 1992; Neugebauer et al. 1993; Nikolajsen et al. 2000; Nikolajsen et al. 1996; Ren et al. 1992; Suzuki et al. 2001; Takahashi et al. 1996; Tseng 1998). The second feature is the dopaminergic agonist action of amantadine (Karobath 1974; Vernier et al. 1969) as illustrated by the inhibition of its uptake (Fletcher and Redfern 1970; Heikkila and Cohen 1972) and an increase of its release (Brown and Redfern 1976; Quack et al. 1995; Stromberg et al. 1970). The results further support the possibility that the activation of the mesolimbic dopaminergic system increases dopamine release within the ACC and diminishes nociception (Saade et al. 1997; Sotres-Bayón et al. 2001). The findings suggest that the main inhibitory effect of amantadine in the ACC is mediated by an interaction with the mesolimbic dopaminergic system. Dopamine D1 and D2 receptor antagonists block the long-term antinociceptive effect produced by the highest dose of amantadine (1000 mM) (Figure 9). Nevertheless, an additional antinociceptive action through the glutamatergic system cannot be discarded. To our knowledge, this is the first study that shows both prophylactic and therapeutic antinociceptive effects of amantadine microinjections into the ACC (López-Avila et al. 2004a). It is important to note that a unique dose of amantadine (200 mg IV) reduced chronic pain (Eisenberg and Pud 1998; Pud et al. 1998) for time periods far longer than the drug's mean life and with minimal secondary effects. Our results suggest that amantadine could be efficient in the reduction of pain by deafferentation.

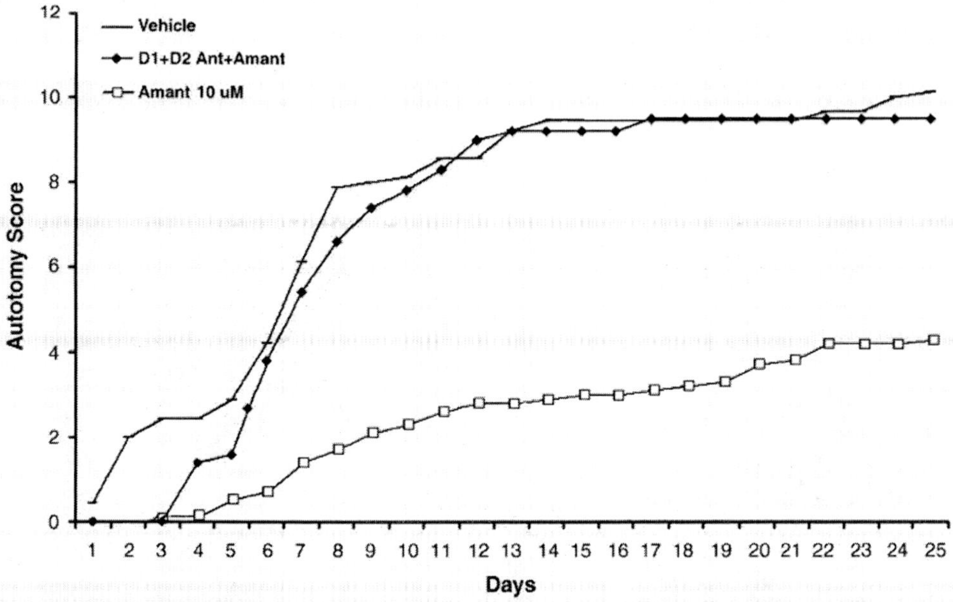

Figure 9. Long-term nociceptive response measured through autotomy score for 25 days. Vehicle (n = 14). Group D1+D2 receptor antagonist + amantadine 1000 uM (n = 10); with a microinjection of a mixture (1 ul) of a D1 receptor antagonist 30 nM (SCH-23390) and a D2 receptor antagonist 300 nM (spiperone); immediately after the microinjection of the mentioned mixture 1 ul of amantadine 2 mM was administered into the ACC. Notice a significant decrease in autotomy score in the amandatine 10 uM group (For the statistical differences between amant 10 uM group and vehicle refer to Figure 8). There were no differences found between groups D1+D2 ant + amant and vehicle.

NOCICEPTIVE RELATED MEMORY AND THE ACC

Structures traditionally associated with the limbic system like the hippocampus, temporal lobe, amygdala, accumbens nuclei and ACC are importantly involved in learning and memory processes (Chapman 1996; Devinsky et al. 1995; Jarrard 1993; Schacter et al. 1989; Setlow et al. 2000; Wan et al. 1999; Wiig and Burwell 1998).

Among the highly relevant brain functions that are related to nociception and pain processing is memory. There is a difference between memory access in terms of evoking knowledge and another one related to pain in which the evocation regards not the knowledge but the aversive alarm condition related to the emotion that regards the pain context in which it was triggered. The mechanisms regarding pain memories are poorly studied in chronic pain states.

Acetylcholine has been classically established as responsible for memory (Drachman and Leavitt 1974). The cingulate cortex, as an important structure of the limbic system, also receives cholinergic projections mainly from the medial septum–diagonal band complex (Gaykema et al. 1990). Moreover, a high density of cholinergic receptors in this brain area has also been demonstrated (Tohyama and Takatsuji 1998). Recent reports show that the cingulate cortex plays a role in postraining memory processing (Farr et al. 2000). Moreover, Devinsky et al. (1995) suggest that the ACC might be related to learning associated with prediction and avoidance of noxious stimuli.

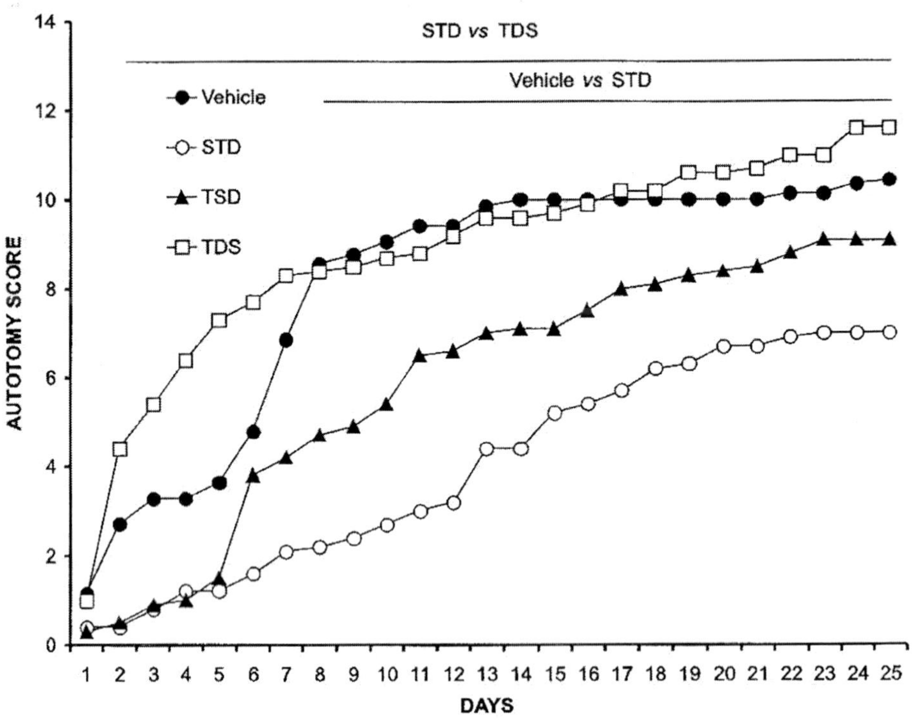

Figure 10. Behavioural nociceptive-related memory response measured as autotomy score along 25 days. All groups were denervated 30 min after thermonociception. Vehicle (n = 14) was microinjected with saline 0.9% into ACC before thermonociception (hind paw immersed in 55 °C water for 20 seconds). Experimental groups (n = 10 each) were injected with scopolamine (10ug in 0.25ul) into the ACC either before thermonociception (STD), between thermonociception and denervation (TSD) or after both manoeuvres (TDS). STD group shows a decreased autotomy score as compared to vehicle and TDS (repeated measured ANOVA, $p < 0.05$). The significant differences between groups per day were established by a Tukey test as a post hoc ($p < 0.05$) (horizontal bars).

In this sense, it was relevant to test if a cholinergic blockade of the ACC is capable of modifying chronic nociception measured as AB. In order to test if the blockade has an effect on the acquisition or maintenance of the nociceptive information an experimental approach was designed. Scopolamine, a cholinergic antagonist, was microinjected into the ACC to test its capability of interfering with memory and learning processes related to chronic nociception. The neuropathic pain model was induced, as in other experimental approaches regarding chronic nociception, by denervation. Also, the nociceptive process was increased by a painful stimulation (Thermonociception) applied 30 minutes prior to denervation in order to enhance AB (Coderre et al. 1986; López-Avila et al. 1999).

The results show a functional relationship between nociception-related memory and ACC in a chronic nociceptive model, which is susceptible of being modified by a blockade of cholinergic transmission (Ortega-Legaspi et al. 2003) (Figure 10).

Sensory nociceptive activity, previous to peripheral deafferentation conditions somatosensory states, particularly painful ones. Clinical evidence shows that the referred pain after amputation (i.e., phantom limb pain), exhibits topological and sensory characteristics similar to the pain experienced previous to amputation, such experiences have been appointed by several authors (Hill et al. 1996; Katz and Melzack 1990; López-Avila et al. 1999; Melzack 1980) as 'pain memory'.

In this context, the ACC has been related to memory processing. Thus, lesions of the cingulum bundle and cingulate cortex impair spatial memory (Aggleton et al. 1995; Dunnett et al. 1990), and lesion of the ACC retarded acquisition of discriminative avoidance learning (Gabriel et al. 1991; Gabriel et al. 1989). Bilateral cingulectomy impairs acquisition and maintenance of avoidance responses (Devinsky et al. 1995). Besides, Farr et al. (2000) demonstrated that functional manipulations with the microinjection of a cholinergic agonist (arecoline) into the ACC had a significant increasing effect on retention test performance while that of an antagonist (scopolamine) diminished the retention in the same test.

The cingulate cortex is a convergence locus where the unpleasant component of nociceptive input is integrated (Coghill et al. 1994; Hsieh et al. 1995; Jones et al. 1991; Rainville et al. 1997; Tuor et al. 2000), as well as the integration of several tasks related to short term and spatial memories (Aggleton et al. 1995; Dunnett et al. 1990; Gaffan 2002; Ragozzino and Kesner 1998). This anatomic and functional convergence allows us to incide in cortical and subcortical levels of the nociceptive integration system, on the regard of highly significant events that trigger a memory process.

With this framework our results show that the microinjection of scopolamine into the ACC, prior to the application of the nociceptive stimulus prevents the acquisition of nociceptive-related memory (Figure 10). However, scopolamine does not modify retention, understood as the conservation of chronic nociception measured by the autotomy score. The fact that the blockade of the muscarinic system after noxious stimulation supports the idea that thermonociceptive stimuli and denervation, previous to a scopolamine microinjection, are determinant to produce or activate a nociceptive-related memory process. This is due to the fact that these stimuli reach the central systems without being blockated by scopolamine. This can be assumed by comparing this fact to the one in which the blockade is applied prior to any noxious stimulation, what is followed by a reduction in the nociceptive-related memory that is measured as a diminished AB. It is important to note that this experimental approach leaves free the nociceptive stimuli transduction and transmission systems, including subcortical and non-frontal cortical structures. This suggests that scopolamine microinjection into the ACC has a direct relationship with the process of acquisition of nociceptive-related memory. Not only does the scopolamine effect in the ACC modify autotomy score, but it also delays the onset of AB in a scheme dependent manner. The present results suggest that nociceptive-related memory processing within the ACC is similar to those traditionally proposed for other processes in which memory is involved. (Ortega-Legaspi et al. 2003).

General Conclusions

There is plenty of historical evidence that the ACC is closely related to the unpleasantness of pain perception. This evidence is mainly supported by the clinical and surgical studies performed in humans (Foltz and White 1962; Hurt and Ballantine 1974). This evidence has recently been further supported by functional imaging techniques such as positron emission tomography and functional magnetic resonance imaging (Jones et al. 1991; Rainville et al. 1997). Although these studies demonstrate the neuroanatomic and functional correlation of the affective component of pain, they do not allow us to understand neurophysiological mechanisms such as the neural pathways, neurotransmitters and receptors involved. The study of affect in regard of the relationship of the ACC to emotional learning can be attributed to the work of Vogt and Devinsky. In this scope, our group has contributed in quantifying chronic pain as an autolesion behaviour and the experimental lesion of the pathways that project to the ACC has become a powerful tool to study the fine mechanisms that involve neurotransmission systems such as the glutamatergic or dopaminergic ones. This is an experimental approach to complex systems that not only involve the already studied ones, but that allows us to further understand the neurotrasmitter dynamics responsible for the affective component of pain integration within the ACC in animals.

The fact that on one hand, the electrical stimulation of the thalamic AM and MD nuclei, which project directly into the ACC through the cingulum bundle and has been proven as a glutamatergic pathway, enhances SIB and on the other the microinjection of an NMDA receptor antagonist (MK-801) diminishes it gives sufficient evidence to support the role of excitatory aminoacids in the genesis of central chronic nociception (Gigg et al. 1992; López-Avila et al. 2004a; Pirot et al. 1994; Torres-López et al. 2000).

Complementary evidence to the above mentioned is the one given by the effect of the electrical stimulation of the VTA, a dopaminergic nucleus that also projects directly to the ACC but through the anterior-medial forebrain bundle, and the microinjection of dopamine into the ACC that both diminishe AB (López-Avila et al. 2004a; Sotres-Bayón et al. 2001).

The ACC is responsible for the integration of the affective component of pain. We propose a double mechanism that activates or inhibits the affective component of pain within the ACC. In this sense, it is relevant to specify using the above mentioned framework the exact mechanisms by which it is activated or inhibited. The activation of this component regards the glutamatergic pathway. On the other hand, the inhibition is regulated by mesolimbic dopaminergic system pathways (Figure 11).

Indeed, all the discussed evidence in this chapter can eventually be used for clinical purposes. It is evident that the use of NMDA receptor antagonists is not suitable for the clinical treatment of chronic pain due to its diversity of functions and the NMDA receptor wide distribution throughout the central nervous system that make a systemic NMDA blockade not operative. The same rationale can be applied to the use of dopaminergic agonist drugs. Given the NMDA receptor antagonist and dopamine release effect of amantadine is that it became a suitable candidate for us to be used in central chronic nociception. In addition, this drug is an Federal Drugs Administration approved drug for the treatment of Parkinson disease (Quinn 1995) which use is operative. In regard of amantadine and central chronic nociception, our experimental evidence shows that the main antinociceptive mechanism of amantadine is its dopaminergic agonism since a selective dopaminergic blockade and amantadine microinjection impairs the effect of amantadine (Figure 9).

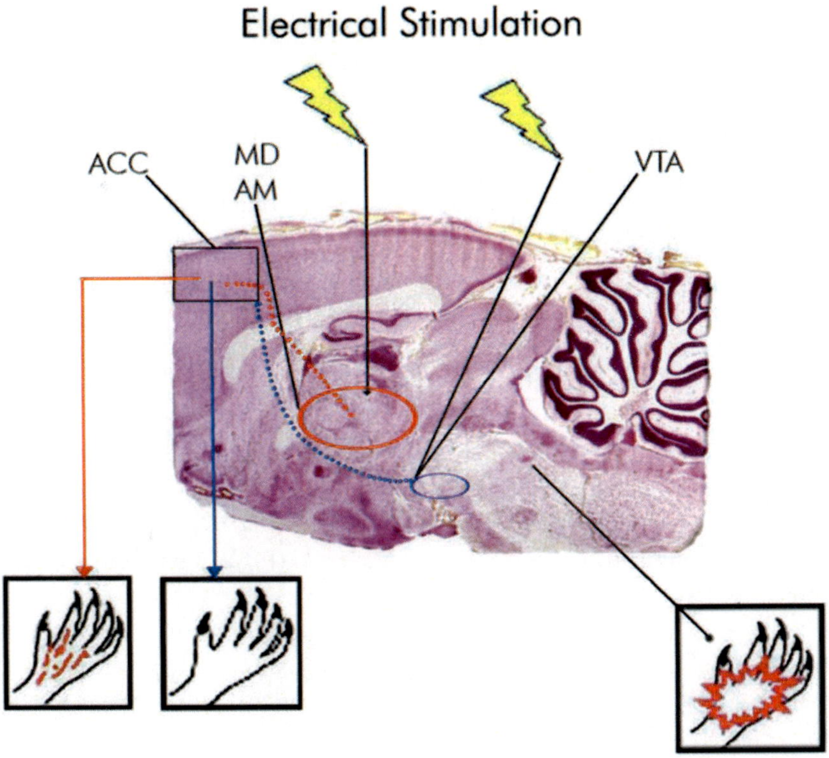

Figure 11. The picture depicts part of the regulatory mechanisms involved in the modulation of the affective component of nociception within the anterior cingulate cortex (ACC). The activation of the glutamatergic pathway that goes from the anteriomedial (AM) and mediodorsal (MD) thalamic nuclei to the ACC through the cingulum bundle enhances the autotomy behaviour triggered by peripheral denervation. The counterpart regulatory system is a dopaminergic one that goes from the ventral tegmental area (VTA) towards the ACC through the medial forebrain bundle and its activation inhibits autotomy behaviour.

Finally, another relevant function of the ACC is the one regarded by nociception-related memory processing. In this sense, the interruption of the nociceptive information acquisition processes within the ACC by the use of a muscarinic inhibition using scopolamine impairs the consolidation of nociception-related memory (Ortega-Legaspi et al. 2003).

Acknowledgements

This research was partially supported by CONACyT FP- 28696M; IMP 3230; Scholarships CONACyT-DGEP UNAM for E.T-L., F.S-B., A.L-A. U.C. and J.M.O-L and Fundación Miguel Alemán for FP.

References

Abbott, F.V. and Melzack, R., Analgesia produced by stimulation of limbic structures and its relation to epileptiform after-discharges, *Experimental Neurology,* 62 (1978) 720-734.

Abercrombie, E.D., Keefe, K.A., DiFrischia, D.S. and Zigmond, M.J., Differential effect of stress on in vivo dopamine release in striatum, nucleus accumbens, and medial frontal cortex, *Journal of Neurochemistry*, 52 (1989) 1655-1658.

Aggleton, J.P., Neave, N., Nagle, S. and Sahgal, A., A comparison of the effects of medial prefrontal, cingulate cortex, and cingulum bundle lesions on tests of spatial memory: evidence of a double dissociation between frontal and cingulum bundle contributions, *The Journal of Neuroscience*, 15 (1995) 7270-7281.

Albe-Fessard, D., Giamberardino, M.A. and Rampin, O., Comparison of different animal models of chronic pain. In: R. Press (Ed.), *Advances in pain research and therapy,* Vol. 13, S. Lipton et al, New York, 1990, pp. 11-27.

Bennett, G.F., Neuropathic pain. In: P.W.a.R. Melzack (Ed.), *Textbook of pain,* Churchill Livingstone, Edingurgh, 1994, pp. 201-224.

Bennett, G.J. and Xie, Y.K., A peripheral mononeuropathy in rat that produces disorders of pain sensation like those seen in man, *Pain*, 33 (1988) 87-107.

Brown, F. and Redfern, P.H., Studies on the mechanism of action of amantadine, *British Journal of Pharmacology*, 58 (1976) 561-567.

Burkey, A.R., Carstens, E. and Jasmin, L., Dopamine reuptake inhibition in the rostral agranular insular cortex produces antinociception, *The Journal of Neuroscience,* 19 (1999) 4169-4179.

Carpenter, K.J. and Dickenson, A.H., NMDA receptors and pain--hopes for novel analgesics, *Regional Anesthesia and Pain Medicine,* 24 (1999) 506-508.

Chang, C. and Shyu, B.C., A fMRI study of brain activations during non-noxious and noxious electrical stimulation of the sciatic nerve of rats, *Brain Research.*, 897 (2001) 71-81.

Chapman, C.R., Limbic processes and the affective dimension of pain, *Progress in Brain Research,* 110 (1996) 63-81.

Coderre, T.J., Grimes, R.W. and Melzack, R., Deafferentation and chronic pain in animals: an evaluation of evidence suggesting autotomy is related to pain, *Pain*, 26 (1986) 61-84.

Coderre, T.J. and Melzack, R., Procedures which increase acute pain sensitivity also increase autotomy, *Experimental Neurology,* 92 (1986) 713-722.

Coghill, R.C., Talbot, J.D., Evans, A.C., Meyer, E., Gjedde, A., Bushnell, M.C. and Duncan, G.H., Distributed processing of pain and vibration by the human brain, *The Journal of Neuroscience*, 14 (1994) 4095-4108.

Davar, G., Hama, A., Deykin, A., Vos, B. and Maciewicz, R., MK-801 blocks the development of thermal hyperalgesia in a rat model of experimental painful neuropathy, *Brain Research*, 553 (1991) 327-330.

Devinsky, O., Morrell, M.J. and Vogt, B.A., Contributions of anterior cingulate cortex to behaviour, *Brain,* 118 (Pt 1) (1995) 279-306.

Dickenson, A.H., Mechanisms of central hypersensitivity: excitatory amino acid mechanisms and their control. The pharmacology of pain, in *Handbook of Experimental Pharmacology* (Dickenson AH and Besson JM eds) Springer Verlag, Berlin (1997) pp 167–210.

Domesick, V.B., The fasciculus cinguli in the rat, *Brain Research.*, 20 (1970) 19-32.

Domesick, V.B., Thalamic relationships of the medial cortex in the rat, *Brain Behavioral Evolution.*, 6 (1972) 457-483.

Dostrovsky, J.O. and Guilbaud, G., Nociceptive responses in medial thalamus of the normal and arthritic rat, *Pain*, 40 (1990) 93-104.

Drachman, D.A. and Leavitt, J., Human memory and the cholinergic system. A relationship to aging?, *Archives of Neurology.*, 30 (1974) 113-121.

Dunnett, S.B., Wareham, A.T. and Torres, E.M., Cholinergic blockade in prefrontal cortex and hippocampus disrupts short-term memory in rats, *Neuroreport*, 1 (1990) 61-64.

Eide, P.K., Clinical Trials of NMDA-Receptor Antagonists as Analgesics. In: Marshall Devor, Michael C. Rowbotham, and Z. Wiesenfeld-Hallin, (Ed.), Proceedings of the 9th World Congress on Pain., *IASP Press*, Seattle, (2000a) pp 817-832.

Eide, P.K., Wind-up and the NMDA receptor complex from a clinical perspective, *European Journal of Pain*, 4 (2000b) 5-15.

Eisenberg, E., LaCross, S. and Strassman, A.M., The effects of the clinically tested NMDA receptor antagonist memantine on carrageenan-induced thermal hyperalgesia in rats, *European Journal of Pharmacology*, 255 (1994) 123-129.

Eisenberg, E. and Pud, D., Can patients with chronic neuropathic pain be cured by acute administration of the NMDA receptor antagonist amantadine?, *Pain,* 74 (1998) 337-339.

Farr, S.A., Uezu, K., Creonte, T.A., Flood, J.F. and Morley, J.E., Modulation of Memory Processing in the Cingulate Cortex of Mice, *Pharmacology, Biochemistry and Behavior,* 65 (2000) 363-368.

Fletcher, E.A. and Redfern, P.H., The effect of amantadine on the uptake of dopamine and noradrenaline by rat brain homogenates, *The Journal of Pharmacy and Pharmacology,* 22 (1970) 957-959.

Foltz, E. and White, L., Pain "relief" by frontal cingulotomy, *Journal Neurosurgery*, 19 (1962) 98-100.

Franklin, K.B., Analgesia and the neural substrate of reward, *Neuroscience and Biobehavioral Reviews*, 13 (1989) 149-154.

Fuster, J.M., The prefrontal cortex: anatomy, physiology and neuropsychology of the frontal lobe, *Lippincott-Raven*, Philadelphia, (1997).

Gabriel, M., Kubota, Y., Sparenborg, S., Straube, K. and Vogt, B.A., Effects of cingulate cortical lesions on avoidance learning and training-induced unit activity in rabbits, *Experimental Brain Research*, 86 (1991) 585-600.

Gabriel, M., Sparenborg, S. and Kubota, Y., Anterior and medial thalamic lesions, discriminative avoidance learning, and cingulate cortical neuronal activity in rabbits, *Experimental Brain Research*, 76 (1989) 441-457.

Gaffan, D., Against memory systems, Philosophical transactions of the Royal Society of London. Series B, *Biological sciences.*, 357 (2002) 1111-1121.

Gao, X., Zhang, Y.Q., Zhang, L.M. and Wu, G.C., Effects of intraplantar injection of carrageenan on central dopamine release, *Brain Research Bulletin*, 54 (2001) 391-394.

Gaykema, R.P., Luiten, P.G., Nyakas, C. and Traber, J., Cortical projection patterns of the medial septum-diagonal band complex, *The Journal of Comparative Neurology*, 293 (1990) 103-124.

Gigg, J., Tan, A.M. and Finch, D.M., Glutamatergic excitatory responses of anterior cingulate neurons to stimulation of the mediodorsal thalamus and their regulation by GABA: an in vivo iontophoretic study, *Cerebral Cortex* , 2 (1992) 477-84.

Gordon, I., Weizman, R. and Rehavi, M., Modulatory effect of agents active in the presynaptic dopaminergic system on the striatal dopamine transporter, *European Journal of Pharmacology*, 298 (1996) 27-30.

Gorea, E. and Lombard, M.C., The possible participation of a dopaminergic system in mutilating behavior in rats with forelimb deafferentation, *Neuroscience Letters*, 48 (1984) 75-80.

Groenewegen, H.J., Organization of the afferent connections of the mediodorsal thalamic nucleus in the rat, related to the mediodorsal-prefrontal topography, *Neuroscience*, 24 (1988) 379-431.

Heikkila, R.E. and Cohen, G., Evaluation of amantadine as a releasing agent or uptake blocker for H 3 -dopamine in rat brain slices, *European Journal of Pharmacology,* 20 (1972) 156-60.

Herrero, J.F., Headley, P.M. and Parsons, C.G., Memantine selectively depresses NMDA receptor-mediated responses of ratspinal neurones in vivo, *Neuroscience Letters*, 165 (1994) 37-40.

Hill, A., Niven, C.A. and Knussen, C., Pain memories in phantom limbs: a case study, *Pain*, 66 (1996) 381-384.

Horikawa, K., Kinjo, N., Stanley, L.C. and Powell, E.W., Topographic organization and collateralization of the projections of the anterior and laterodorsal thalamic nuclei to cingulate areas 24 and 29 in the rat, *Neurosci Research.*, 6 (1988) 31-44.

Hsieh, J.C., Belfrage, M., Stone-Elander, S., Hansson, P. and Ingvar, M., Central representation of chronic ongoing neuropathic pain studied by positron emission tomography, *Pain,* 63 (1995) 225-236.

Hsu, M.M. and Shyu, B.C., Electrophysiological study of the connection between medial thalamus and anterior cingulate cortex in the rat, *Neuroreport*, 8 (1997) 2701-2707.

Hurt, R.W. and Ballantine, H.T., Stereotactic anterior cingulate lesions for persistent pain: a report on 68 cases, *Clinical Neurosurgery*, 21 (1974) 334-351.

Jarrard, L.E., On the role of the hippocampus in learning and memory in the rat, *Behavioral and Neural Biology*, 60 (1993) 9-26.

Jones, A.K., Brown, W.D., Friston, K.J., Qi, L.Y. and Frackowiak, R.S., Cortical and subcortical localization of response to pain in man using positron emission tomography, Philosophical transactions of the Royal Society of London. Series B, *Biological sciences.*, 244 (1991) 39-44.

Jones, A.K. and Derbyshire, S.W.G., Positron Emission Tomography as a Tool for Understanding the Cerebral Processing of Pain. In: J. Boivie, P. Hansson and U.

Lindblom (Eds.), Touch, Temperature, and Pain in Health and Disease: Mechanisms and Assessments., *IASP Press*, Seattle, (1993) pp 491-520.

Karobath, M.E., Amantadine and D-145, an amantadine derivative, do not effect dopamine sensitive adenylate cyclase from the caudate-putamen of the rat brain, *European Journal of Pharmacology,* 28 (1974) 376-378.

Katz, J. and Melzack, R., Pain 'memories' in phantom limbs: review and clinical observations, *Pain,* 43 (1990) 319-336.

Khandwala, H., Hodge, E. and Loomis, C.W., Comparable dose-dependent inhibition of AP-7 sensitive strychnine-induced allodynia and paw pinch-induced nociception by mexiletine in the rat, *Pain*, 72 (1997) 299-308.

Kim, S.H. and Chung, J.M., An experimental model for peripheral neuropathy produced by segmental spinal nerve ligation in the rat, *Pain*, 50 (1992) 355-363.

Kornhuber, J., Bormann, J., Hubers, M., Rusche, K. and Riederer, P., Effects of the 1-amino-adamantanes at the MK-801-binding site of the NMDA-receptor-gated ion channel: a human postmortem brain study, *European Journal of Pharmacology*, 206 (1991) 297-300.

Kornhuber, J., Quack, G., Danysz, W., Jellinger, K., Danielczyk, W., Gsell, W. and Riederer, P., Therapeutic brain concentration of the NMDA receptor antagonist amantadine, *Neuropharmacology,* 34 (1995) 713-721.

Krettek, J.E. and Price, J.L., The cortical projections of the mediodorsal nucleus and adjacent thalamic nuclei in the rat, *The Journal of Comparative Neurology*, 171 (1977) 157-191.

Kristensen, J.D., Svensson, B. and Gordh, T., The NMDA-receptor antagonist CPP abolishes neurogenic 'wind-up pain' after intrathecal administration in humans, *Pain,* 51 (1992) 249-253.

Levitt, M., Dysesthesias and self-mutilation in humans and subhumans: a review of clinical and experimental studies, *Brain Research*, 357 (1985) 247-290.

López-Avila, A., Coffeen, U., Ortega-Legaspi, J.M., del Angel, R. and Pellicer, F., Dopamine and NMDA systems modulate long-term nociception in the rat anterior cingulate cortex, *Pain*, 111 (2004a) 136-143.

López-Avila, A., Rodriguez-Manzo, G., Coffeen, U., del Angel, R. and Pellicer, F., Self-injury behaviour induced by intraplantar carrageenan infiltration: a model of tonic nociception, *Brain Research Protocols*., 13 (2004b) 37-44.

López-Avila, A., Sotres-Bayon, F., del Angel, R. and Pellicer, F., Time span between nociceptive stimulus and denervation modifies autotomy behavior in rat, *Analgesia*, 4 (1999) 475-478.

Luger, T.J., Lorenz, I.H., Grabner-Weiss, C. and Hayashi, T., Effect of the NMDA-antagonist, MK 801, on benzodiazepine-opioid interactions at the spinal and supraspinal level in rats, *British Journal of Pharmacology*, 114 (1995) 1097-1103.

Lutfy, K., Cai, S.X., Woodward, R.M. and Weber, E., Antinociceptive effects of NMDA and non-NMDA receptor antagonists in the tail flick test in mice, *Pain*, 70 (1997) 31-40.

Ma, Q.P., Zhou, Y. and Han, J.S., Electroacupuncture accelerated the expression of c-Fos protooncogene in dopaminergic neurons in the ventral tegmental area of the rat, *International Journal Of Neuroscience,* 70 (1993) 217-222.

Magnusson, J.E. and Vaccarino, A.L., Reduction of autotomy following peripheral neurectomy by a single injection of bupivacaine into the cingulum bundle of rats, *Brain* Research, 723 (1996) 214-217.

Mantz, J., Milla, C., Glowinski, J. and Thierry, A.M., Differential effects of ascending neurons containing dopamine and noradrenaline in the control of spontaneous activity and of evoked responses in the rat prefrontal cortex, *Neuroscience*, 27 (1988) 517-526.

Mao, J., Price, D.D., Mayer, D.J., Lu, J. and Hayes, R.L., Intrathecal MK-801 and local nerve anesthesia synergistically reduce nociceptive behaviors in rats with experimental peripheral mononeuropathy, *Brain Research,* 576 (1992) 254-262.

Mayer, D.J. and Liebeskind, J.C., Pain reduction by focal electrical stimulation of the brain: an anatomical and behavioral analysis, *Brain Research.*, 68 (1974) 73-93.

Mayer, D.J. and Price, D.D., Central nervous system mechanisms of analgesia, *Pain*, 2 (1976) 379-404.

Melzack, R., Psychologic aspects of pain, *Research publications - Association for Research in Nervous and Mental Disease.*, 58 (1980) 143-54.

Morelli, M., Fenu, S., Pinna, A., Cozzolino, A., Carta, A. and Di Chiara, G., "Priming" to dopamine agonist-induced contralateral turning as a model of non-associative sensitization to the expression of the post-synaptic dopamine message, *Behavioral Pharmacology.*, 4 (1993) 389-397.

Morgan, M.J. and Franklin, K.B., 6-Hydroxydopamine lesions of the ventral tegmentum abolish D-amphetamine and morphine analgesia in the formalin test but not in the tail flick test, *Brain Research*, 519 (1990) 144-149.

Nasstrom, J., Karlsson, U. and Berge, O.G., Systemic or intracerebroventricular injection of NMDA receptor antagonists attenuates the antinociceptive activity of intrathecally administered NMDA receptor antagonists, *Brain Research*, 623 (1993) 47-55.

Neugebauer, V., Kornhuber, J., Lucke, T. and Schaible, H.G., The clinically available NMDA receptor antagonist memantine is antinociceptive on rat spinal neurones, *Neuroreport,* 4 (1993) 1259-1262.

Nikolajsen, L., Gottrup, H., Kristensen, A.G. and Jensen, T.S., Memantine (a N-methyl-D-aspartate receptor antagonist) in the treatment of neuropathic pain after amputation or surgery: a randomized, double-blinded, cross-over study, *Anesthesia and Analgesia,* 91 (2000) 960-966.

Nikolajsen, L., Hansen, C.L., Nielsen, J., Keller, J., Arendt_Nielsen, L. and Jensen, T.S., The effect of ketamine on phantom pain: a central neuropathic disorder maintained by peripheral input, *Pain,* 67 (1996) 69-77.

Ortega-Legaspi, J.M., López-Avila, A., Coffeen, U., del Angel, R. and Pellicer, F., Scopolamine into the anterior cingulate cortex diminishes nociception in a neuropathic pain model in the rat: an interruption of 'nociception-related memory acquisition'?, *European Journal of Pain.*, 7 (2003) 425-429.

Papez, J.W., A proposed mechanism of emotion, Archives of Neurology and Psychiatry, 38 (1937) 725-743.

Pellicer, F., López-Avila, A. and Torres-López, E., Electric stimulation of the cingulum bundle precipitates onset of autotomy induced by inflammation in rat, *European Journal of Pain*, 3 (1999) 287-293.

Pirot, S., Jay, T.M., Glowinski, J. and Thierry, A.M., Anatomical and electrophysiological evidence for an excitatory amino acid pathway from the thalamic mediodorsal nucleus to the prefrontal cortex in the rat, *The European Journal of Neuroscience,* 6 (1994) 1225-1234.

Pud, D., Eisenberg, E., Spitzer, A., Adler, R., Fried, G. and Yarnitsky, D., The NMDA receptor antagonist amantadine reduces surgical neuropathic pain in cancer patients: a double blind, randomized, placebo controlled trial, *Pain*, 75 (1998) 349-354.

Quack, G., Hesselink, M., Danysz, W. and Spanagel, R., Microdialysis studies with amantadine and memantine on pharmacokinetics and effects on dopamine turnover, *Journal of Neural Transmission*. Suppl., 46 (1995) 97-105.

Quinn, N., Drug treatment of Parkinson's disease, *British Medical Journal*, 310 (1995) 575-9.

Ragozzino, M.E. and Kesner, R.P., The effects of muscarinic cholinergic receptor blockade in the rat anterior cingulate and Prelimbic/Infralimbic cortices on spatial working memory, *Neurobiology Learning and Memory*., 69 (1998) 241-257.

Rainville, P., Duncan, G.H., Price, D.D., Carrier, B. and Bushnell, M.C., Pain affect encoded in human anterior cingulate but not somatosensory cortex, *Science*, 277 (1997) 968-971.

Ren, K., Hylden, J.L., Williams, G.M., Ruda, M.A. and Dubner, R., The effects of a non-competitive NMDA receptor antagonist, MK-801, on behavioral hyperalgesia and dorsal horn neuronal activity in rats with unilateral inflammation, *Pain*, 50 (1992) 331-344.

Rinaldi, P.C., Young, R.F., Albe-Fessard, D. and Chodakiewitz, J., Spontaneous neuronal hyperactivity in the medial and intralaminar thalamic nuclei of patients with deafferentation pain, *Journal of Neurosurgery*, 74 (1991) 415-421.

Saade, N.E., Atweh, S.F., Bahuth, N.B. and Jabbur, S.J., Augmentation of nociceptive reflexes and chronic deafferentation pain by chemical lesions of either dopaminergic terminals or midbrain dopaminergic neurons, *Brain Research*, 751 (1997) 1-12.

Sarkis, D., Souteyrand, J.P. and Albe-Fessard, D., Self-stimulation in the ventral tegmental area suppresses self-mutilation in rats with forelimb deafferentiation, *Neuroscience Letters*, 44 (1984) 199-204.

Schacter, G.B., Yang, C.R., Innis, N.K. and Mogenson, G.J., The role of the hippocampal-nucleus accumbens pathway in radial-arm maze performance, *Brain Research*, 494 (1989) 339-349.

Seltzer, Z., Dubner, R. and Shir, Y., A novel behavioral model of neuropathic pain disorders produced in rats by partial sciatic nerve injury, *Pain*, 43 (1990) 205-218.

Setlow, B., Roozendaal, B. and McGaugh, J.L., Involvement of a basolateral amygdala complex-nucleus accumbens pathway in glucocorticoid-induced modulation of memory consolidation, *The European Journal of Neuroscience*, 12 (2000) 367-375.

Shibata, H. and Kato, A., Topographic relationship between anteromedial thalamic nucleus neurons and their cortical terminal fields in the rat, *Neuroscience Research*, 17 (1993) 63-69.

Sikes, R.W. and Vogt, B.A., Nociceptive neurons in area 24 of rabbit cingulate cortex, *Journal Of Neurophysiology*, 68 (1992) 1720-1732.

Sotres-Bayón, F., Torres-Lopez, E., López-Avila, A., del Angel, R. and Pellicer, F., Lesion and electrical stimulation of the ventral tegmental area modify persistent nociceptive behavior in the rat, *Brain Research*, 898 (2001) 342-349.

Stone, T.W., Responses of neurones in the cerebral cortex and caudate nucleus to amantadine, amphetamine and dopamine, *British Journal of Pharmacology*, 56 (1976) 101-110.

Stromberg, U., Svensson, T.H. and Waldeck, B., On the mode of action of amantadine, *The Journal of Pharmacy and Pharmacology*, 22 (1970) 959-962.

Suzuki, R., Matthews, E.A. and Dickenson, A.H., Comparison of the effects of MK-801, ketamine and memantine on responses of spinal dorsal horn neurones in a rat model of mononeuropathy, *Pain*, 91 (2001) 101-109.

Takahashi, T., Yamashita, H., Zhang, Y.X. and Nakamura, S., Inhibitory effect of MK-801 on amantadine-induced dopamine release in the rat striatum, *Brain Research Bulletin*, 41 (1996) 363-367.

Thierry, A.M., Tassin, J.P., Blanc, G. and Glowinski, J., Selective activation of mesocortical DA system by stress, *Nature*, 263 (1976) 242-244.

Tohyama, M., *The acetylcholinergic system* In: Tohyama, M., and Takatsuji, K., (Eds) Atlas of neuroactive substances and their receptors in the rat, Oxford University Press, 1998, pp 66-95.

Toide, K., Effects of amantadine on dopaminergic neurons in discrete regions of the rat brain, *Pharmaceutical Research,* 7 (1990) 670-672.

Torres-López, E., del Angel, R. and Pellicer, F., Thalamic anteromedial and mediodorsal nuclei stimulation enhances the self-injury behavior induced by an inflammatory process in the rat, *Analgesia*, 5 (2000) 67-73.

Tseng, S.H., Suppression of autotomy by N-methyl-D-aspartate receptor antagonist (MK-801) in the rat, *Neuroscience Letters*, 240 (1998) 17-20.

Tuor, U.I., Malisza, K., Foniok, T., Papadimitropoulos, R., Jarmasz, M., Somorjai, R. and Kozlowski, P., Functional magnetic resonance imaging in rats subjected to intense electrical and noxious chemical stimulation of the forepaw, *Pain,* 87 (2000) 315-324.

Vaccarino, A.I. and Melzack, R., The role of the cingulum bundle in self-mutilation following peripheral neurectomy in the rat, *Experimental Neurology*, 111 (1991) 131-134.

Vernier, V.G., Harmon, J.B., Stump, J.M., Lynes, T.E., Marvel, J.P. and Smith, D.H., The toxicologic and pharmacologic properties of amantadine hydrochloride, *Toxicology and Applied Pharmacology*, 15 (1969) 642-665.

Vogt, B.A., Finch, D.M. and Olson, C.R., Functional heterogeneity in cingulate cortex: the anterior executive and posterior evaluative regions, *Cerebral Cortex.,* 5 (1992) 435-443.

Wall, P.D., Devor, M., Inbal, R., Scadding, J.W., Schonfeld, D., Seltzer, Z. and Tomkiewicz, M.M., Autotomy following peripheral nerve lesions: experimental anaesthesia dolorosa, *Pain*, 7 (1979) 103-111.

Wan, H., Aggleton, J.P. and Brown, M.W., Different contributions of the hippocampus and perirhinal cortex to recognition memory, *The Journal of Neuroscience,* 19 (1999) 1142-1148.

Wiig, K.A. and Burwell, R.D., Memory impairment on a delayed non-matching-to-position task after lesions of the perirhinal cortex in the rat, *Behavioral Neuroscience*, 112 (1998) 827-838.

Yamamura, H., Iwata, K., Tsuboi, Y., Toda, K., Kitajima, K., Shimizu, N., Nomura, H., Hibiya, J., Fujita, S. and Sumino, R., Morphological and electrophysiological properties of ACCx nociceptive neurons in rats, *Brain Research*, 735 (1996) 83-92.

Zeltser, R. and Seltzer, Z., A practical guide for the use of animal models in the study of neuropathic pain. In: J. Boivie, P. Hansson and U. Lindblom (Eds.), *Touch, Temperature, and Pain in Health and Disease: Mechanisms and Assessments, Vol. 3,* IASP Press, Seattle, 1994, pp. 295- 338.

Zimmerman, M., Ethical guidelines for investigations of experimental pain in conscious animals, *Pain*, 16 (1983) 109-110.

In Frontiers in Pain Research
Editor: Alexendre Lucas, pp.157-176
ISBN 1-59454-828-5

Chapter 8

PAIN AND CELEBRATING NEW LIFE: WOMEN GIVING BIRTH

Lynn Clark Callister*
Brigham Young University College of Nursing, Provo, UT

ABSTRACT

Childbirth provides the paradoxical circle of both pain and joy with physical, emotional, cognitive, and spiritual dimensions. Complex factors influence childbirth pain. This chapter reports on two decades of qualitative cross cultural studies of childbearing women and a review of the literature focusing on attitudes, perceptions, and meaning of the pain associated with giving birth, pain related behaviors, coping mechanisms for dealing with childbirth pain, and management f the pain of childbirth. Implications for clinical practice and future research are identified.

INTRODUCTION

Pain can be both positive and/or negative, and experiencing pain may be fundamental in fostering personal growth (Aldrich & Eccleston, 2000). Childbirth is a significant life event representing a major pain experience that accompanies the normal physiologic process of giving birth" (Callister, Khalaf, Semenic, et al, 2003). For some first time expectant mothers, giving birth may be their "first experience with significant physical pain" (Lowe, 2002, p. S20). Assumptions about childbirth pain are found in Table 1.

The pain of childbirth has been defined as "a unique and complex sensory and affective experience that differs from the acute or chronic pain of disease, trauma, surgical, or medical procedures" (Callister, Khalaf, Semenic, et al, 2003, p. 145). Unlike other types of pain, it is important to note that, "Birth is characterized by pain but also by the most positive of life events—[creating] a new life" (Niven & Gijsbers,. 1996, p. 131).

Table 1. Assumptions About Pain

- Pain is REAL
- Pain and the pain response are intensely personal
- Pain holds different meanings
- Different pain holds different meanings for the same person
- Pain is a recognized part of giving birth
- Pain has the potential for causing distress or damage
- Pain is not the opposite of comfort
- Pain that is established is more difficult to manage than early pain
- Pain fear is powerful
- The best source of pain information is the individual
- Long term recall of labor pain is vivid but not entirely accurate
- Pain is not predictive of satisfaction with childbirth

Source: Bianchi & Adams, 2004; Corbett & Callister, 2000; Goodman, Mackey & Tavakoli, 2004; Jimenez, 1998, Maternity Center Association, 2002; Matthews & Callister, 2004; Niven & Murphy-Black, 2000; Petree & Walsch, 2001; Simkin, 1991

Factors which influence childbirth pain include the intensity and duration of contractions, cervical dilation (degree of and rate), perineal distention, maternal age/physical condition/parity, fetal size and position, length of labor, obstetrical interventions, mode of birth (Cesarean or non-instrumental/instrumental vaginal birth), and factors such as personal beliefs, cultural expectations, feelings of control, perceptions of discomfort and pain, fear, anxiety, and expectations for the birth experience (Goodman, Mackey & Tavakoli, 2004; Green & Baston, 2003; Hodnett, 2002; Jimenez, 2000; Maclean, McDermott & May, 2000; Mander, 1998; Nystedt, Hogberg & Lundman, 2005; Petree & Walsch, 2001; VandeVusse, 1999; Waldenstrom, 1999). During cervical dilation, pain results from distention of the lower uterus and dilation. During descent of the fetus, there is an increase in somatic pain resulting from distention and traction on pelvic structures around the vagina. One woman described it in this way,

> When she [the baby] crowned there was really an intense pain that I wasn't prepared for at all. It was burning and stretching. I can imagine why some women feel like they are being split in half.

This report of two decades of qualitative research with childbearing women and a review of the literature will focus on attitudes, perceptions, and meaning of the pain associated with giving birth, pain related behaviors, coping mechanisms for dealing with childbirth pain, and management of the pain of childbirth. Implications for clinical practice and future research are identified.

* Lynn_callister@byu.edu; (801) 422-3227; Fax (801) 422-0536

ATTITUDES, PERCEPTIONS OF, AND MEANING OF CHILDBIRTH PAIN

Perceptions of childbirth pain vary widely. Women with an understanding of the processes of labor may consider pain to be a positive sign of progress toward giving birth. Women with an understanding that the pain of childbirth is a non-threatening life experience to be mastered may also view pain differently than those who perceive giving birth as a potentially dangerous event fraught with risk (Lowe, 2002). Women espousing the mastery model of childbirth may experience great satisfaction as they negotiate a challenging life event, regardless of the pain experienced (Bianchi, 1996; Capik, 1998). This was expressed by one mother who gave birth unmedicated,

> It was great. I felt like a hero—"Hey, I made it!" Nothing about it was easy, absolutely nothing. But there is a great feeling of the last minute of pushing, when [the baby] finally slides out. There is no such feeling in the world (Callister, Semenic & Foster, 1999, p. 286).

According to an anthropologist, "Every culture ritualizes birth, as it is one of the most significant rites of passage in the social life of mother and child" (Davis-Floyd, 1986, p. 121). Childbirth pain is also culturally bound (Lasch, 2000; Nayak, Shiflet, Eshun, et al, 2000; Weber, 1996). "The perception of pain and behaviors associated with pain are influenced by the sociocultural context of the [woman] experiencing pain" (Callister, 2003, p.211; Callister, 1995, 2001, 2006; Callister, Lauri, Vehvailnen-Julkunen, 2000; Callister, Vehvailinen-Julkunen & Lauri, 1996). In The Netherlands, many women give birth at home with minimal interventions (Schrim, Tobi & Vandenberg, 2002; Johnson & Callister in review; van der Hulst, van Teijlingen, Bonsel, Eskes, et al, 2004). Women giving birth in Finland expect pain as part of the childbirth process and describe working with the contractions rather than fighting against the intensity of the experience, citing the Finnish proverb, "Life is more than a dance on a bed of roses" (Callister, Vehvailinen-Julkunen & Lauri, 2001). Women giving birth in Guatemala and Jordan speak of the bittersweet paradox of giving birth (Callister & Vega, 1998; Khalaf & Callister, 1997). This paradox has been described by women giving birth in the People's Republic of China as *xianku houtian* (first bitter, then sweet) (Kartchner & Callister, 2003). The paradox of pain, suffering, and comfort in Swedish women's childbirth experiences has been documented (Lundgren & Dahlberg, 1998). One woman in their study described it this way, *"It was hell, and a little more, but felt good anyway"* (p.108). Negative and positive feelings about childbirth pain can coexist, and "a positive experience does not preclude pain and distress" (Waldenstrom, Berg, Olsson, et al, 1996, p. 152). One Russian mother who gave birth unmedicated said,

> During contractions I was only thinking, 'is it possible to love the child after this?' But when she was born and lying on chest, she looked at me. At that time I forgot all the pain (Callister, Getmanenko, Garvrish, Eugenevna, Vladiminov, Turkina & Lassetter, in press).

Factors associated with women's perceptions of birth as being traumatic include inadequate pain relief, feelings of powerlessness, lack of support, lack of control, and unmet expectations which may result in post-traumatic stress disorder (Beck, 2004a, b; Creedy, Shochet & Horsfall, 2000; Czarnocka & Slade, 2000; Fowles, 1998; Melender & Lauri, 2001; Soet, Breck & Dilorio, 2003; Waldenstrom, Hildingsson, Rubertsson & Radestad, 2004;

Waldenstrom, 2004). An interesting work compared pain intensity and pain catastrophizing. Researchers concluded that labor pain catastrophiziing rather than the intensity of labor pain was predictive of postpartum mood disorders and social functioning (Ferber, Granot & Zimmer, 2005). Pain catastrophizing included focusing on the pain, exaggerating the negative consequences of the pain, and feelings of helplessness during the pain experience.

Some women in the studies cited above felt that epidural analgesia/anesthesia detracted from the quality of their birth experience. One woman in a related study reported,

> I had my first baby [in a way] I view as traditional, where the doctor was in control and he encouraged me to have an epidural. It was such a frightening experience. Afterwards I thought, "This isn't childbirth. There's got to be more to it than just laying there with a numb body (Callister, 1994, p. 254).

Some women express concern about potential side effects associated with epidural analgesia, such as this first time mother,

> I had a very easy labor. In fact, I remember being surprised that my pain wasn't worse. [Women] say it's so awful and you're gonna have to have an epidural. Well, the whole idea of an epidural really scared me bad. I just do not like the thought of someone putting a needle in my spine. I was determined that I would only use it if absolutely necessary. But it wasn't that bad. Yea, it hurt a lot but it wasn't as bad as I had made it out to be. It was really a lot better than I thought (Callister, Khalaf, Semenic, et al, 2003, p. 147).

Other women expressed relief at having epidural analgesia, such as this mother,

> After I received the epidural, I felt relaxed and actually excited about my birth. The epidural made me feel more comfortable and calmer.

The absence of pain is not necessarily equated with positive outcomes from childbirth. In a systematic review of pain and women's satisfaction with the experience of childbirth, Hodnett (2002, p. 169) concluded that, "Pain and pain relief do not play major roles in satisfaction with the childbirth experience, unless expectations regarding either are unmet." This is supported by British researchers who concluded that, "A painful birth is just as likely to have a positive evaluation as a pain free one; reduction of pain [alone] will do nothing to promote a generally positive childbirth experience" (Salmon, Miller & Drew, 1990, p. 258). One multiparous woman said,

> When I was in labor, the pain was something I had never experienced in the whole world. Right before the baby was born there was more pain than I could think of, but then I saw the baby there was a happiness more than I could think of (Callister, Khalaf, Semenic, et al, 2003, p. 148).

In a study of women who had indicated a preference for an unmedicated birth who subsequently had epidural analgesia, Kanna and associates (2001) noted that 88% of their sample who had epidurals reported being less satisfied with their birth experience despite lower intensity of pain. In other work, women have reported feeling lack of control related to numbness of their legs and being unable to move (Fowles, 1998).

One woman having an unmedicated birth framed her experience as a time of personal growth and self actualization,

> I think I have a right to feel good about myself. In a way, this birth is helping me to accept myself—both the limitations and the capabilities. Accepting myself is the other side of the coin of accepting the pain. I have a sense that for me this has considerable significance (Bergum 1989, p. 81).

Another woman articulated her experience with an unmedicated birth,

> I would never have wanted it any other way. It gave me confidence and strength. I was able to deal with the pain, to confront and overcome. NowI know that I can deal with it—and that is useful in encountering other painful things (Bergum, 1989, p. 1989)

In a phenomenological study of the meaning of childbirth pain, pain was seen as an essential component of giving birth characterized as being both positive and negative (Lundgren & Dahlber, 1998). The meaning of pain has described as multi-facted, like peeling away the layers of an onion to discover hidden and complex meanings (Mander, 1996, 2000). A Jewish mother described her experience in this way:

> Once he came out, I felt exhilarated. I couldn't believe that the baby came, that the pain would be over. I was crying and laughing at the same time from happiness(Callister, et al, 2003, p. 147).

Women have described the importance of feeling in control, of actively participating in giving birth, of having a voice in childbirth care decisions, and a birthing environment characterized by respect and support (Callister, 1994; Fowles, 1998; Waldenstrom, 2004). In postpartum women, feelings of personal control had a positive impact on women's satisfaction with pain relief during labor (McCrea & Wright, 1999; Wright, McCrea, Stringer, et al, 2000). Lowe's work over two decades has documented that there is an inverse relationship between a woman's confidence in her ability to cope and perceived pain (2000, 2004). This thought has been expressed,

> In the United States, there seems to be a popular belief that labor pain is bad, and the parturient should be relieved of her pain as possible. These beliefs seem paradoxic in a society that celebrates individuals who endure great pain and distress in the pursuit of mountain peaks or completion of a marathon race. Childbirth has deep significance for everyone—it is a profound physiologic, psychosocial, and spiritual event. It is this context of the experience of childbirth that dries some women to experience all of labor, even it's pain…as only one component of the totality of the woman's labor and birth experience (Lowe, 2002, S23).

Having a sense of control is emerging as a significant variable in childbearing women. In the literature, there is currently not a universal conceptualization of control. Being involved in decision making (or being in control of what interventions are applied) is the most frequently addressed type of external control. Internal control has do to with control of behavior during labor and birth and a sense of control while experiencing contractions. Two major threats to a woman's sense of internal control are pain and the side effects of pain relief.

In a study of the relationship between self-efficacy and childbirth fears in first time expectant mothers, women with a high level of fear also had higher levels of learned helplessness, chance health locus of control, powerful others health locus of control, and significantly lower self control and self-efficacy (Lowe, 2000).Worry during pregnancy about the pain of labor is an important predictor of satisfaction with childbirth in first time mothers (Green & Baston, 2003). These researchers concluded that what strategies are employed to help women deal with the pain of childbirth has an effect on internal control, and that the extent to which professionals share decision making power affects external control (Green & Baston, 2003). These findings are supported in a study of women having unmedicated births (Hardin & Buckner, 2004) indicating that women felt the ability to control their bodies during labor and the ability to influence the birthing environment contributed to a positive birth experience.

Pain Related Behaviors

Reasons for an emotive response to pain include fear of pain, desire for help and fear of not receiving it, a sense of losing dignity, fear of losing control, and fear of side effects from pain medication. Pain related behaviors are also culturally bound, and in some women there may be a perceived exorcism of pain through the act of crying out (Luckmann, 1999). In other cultures such as among Asian and Native American women, women focus inward and appear stoic. Women during transition describe losing the ability to keep things in perspective, feeling that they are no longer able to keep "on top" of their contractions, shaking uncontrollably, feeling confused, feeling irritated and wanting to go home (Mander, 1998).

Coping Mechanisms for Dealing with Childbirth Pain

A variety of coping mechanisms may be utilized to manage the pain of labor and birth.

A spiritual lifestyle is a source of coping for some childbearing women (Callister, 1992; Callister, Khalaf, Semenic, et al, 2003; Callister, Semenic & Foster, 1999; Callister & Vega, 1998; Semenic, Callister & Feldman, 2004). One woman expressed her feelings this way,

> When it got to the worst part of the pain that's when you look up to heaven for God's help. Sometimes during the labor I would cry out in pain and say, "Jesus, help me." I felt like God was saving me as I gave birth" (Callister, Khalaf, Semenic, et al, 2003, p. 149).

Creating a birth plan may be an important strategy for women preparing to give birth and manage their pain. There may be benefits to creating a birth plan as related to reduction of fear and pain (Lundgren, Berg, & Lindmark, 2003). One nurse described it in this way,

> A woman sees the birth plan as a way of being empowered. If a woman comes in with a framework of what she wants, she's tried to do her homework. She's tried to figure out what she should and shouldn't do…I like that" (James, Simpson & Knox, 2003, p. 820).

Women should be encouraged to keep their options for pain management open rather than being rigid and inflexible on the goal to have an unmedicated birth versus the desire to have epidural analgesia at the first twinge of pain (Petree & Walsch, 2001). Women describe the importance of feeling in control, of actively participating in giving birth, of having a voice in childbirth care decisions, having their expectations met, and a birthing environment characterized by respect and support (Callister, 1994; Goodman, Mackey & Tavakoli, 2004; Lavender, Walkinshaw & Walton, 1999).

In a landmark work by Poore and Foster (1985) differences were identified in women who were either unmedicated or received epidural analgesia/anesthesia in their sense of control and active participation in childbirth care decisions. In a study of 17 women who gave birth unmedicated, study participants reported a high level of satisfaction with their birth experience. These women identified feeling in control and being supported as the major factors contributing to a positive birth experience (Hardin & Buckner, 2004).

Management of Childbirth Pain

According to Joint Commission accreditation standards (JCAHO, 2003), women have the right to effective pain management during labor and birth. Pain management includes a multiple of strategies, not just the use of pharmacologic agents (Caton, Frolich & Euliano, 2002; Caton, Corry, Frigoletto, et al, 2002). It should be noted that in those women being induced the pain experience may be challenging from the beginning, rather than increasing in intensity over time. This makes it particularly difficult for women receiving oxytocin to have an unmedicated birth. One woman said about being induced, *"The pain is the most intense I have ever experienced. It is all consuming and as I was induced appears to never let go"* (Green, Coupland & Kitzinger, 1998, p. 83).

Epidural Analgesia/Anesthesia and Other Pharmacological Methods

Epidural analgesia/anesthesia provides effective pain relief and is widely used in the United States for management of the pain of childbirth. Guidelines for the nursing care for women receiving epidural analgesia/anesthesia have been generated (Association of Womens Health, Obstetric, and Neonatal Nurses [AWHONN], 2001).

However, in a Cochrane review of 11 studies and another systematic review, there was evidence of potential side effects including increased length of first and second stage labor, the need for augmentation with oxytocin, increased fetal malposition, and increased instrumental vaginal birth (Enkin, Keirse, Neilson, et al, 2000; Howell, 2004; Leeman, Fontaine, King, et al, 2003a; Leighton & Halpern, 2002; Lieberman & Donoghue, 2002; Mayberry, Clemmens & De, 2002; Thacker & Stroup, 2002). Only one study documented the effects of epidural analgesia on neonatal behavior, breastfeeding, and maternal-infant bonding (Kardong-Edgren, 1999). Longitudinal studies are needed to determine the maternal and neonatal effects of epidurals. It has been purported that,

> In normal birth, there are complex hormonal shifts that help labor progress and facilitate birth. The laboring woman produces natural endorphins that help her manage the pain of labor...Epidural analgesia numbs the sensations of birth and the production of natural endorphins ceases as a result of the disruption of the hormonal feedback system (Torvaldsen, Roberts, Bell, et al, 2004).

Further, this meta-analysis of five randomized clinical trials found that discontinuing the epidural late in labor was associated with a statistically significant increase in inadequate pain relief (Torvaldsen, Roberts, Bell, et al, 2004). Further research is needed on the acceptability of the practice of letting the epidural "wear off" on maternal satisfaction with the birth experience.

Other pharmacological methods include parenteral opiates, paracervical blocks, and nitrous oxide. Parenteral opiods provide less effective pain relief and such neonatal effects may include respiratory depression, neurobehavioral effects such as decreased alertness, ineffective sucking which delays effective breastfeeding (Bricker & Lavender, 2002; Leeman, Fontaine & King, et al, 2003a). Nitrous oxide is seldom used in the United States for childbirth pain and produces poor recall of the birth experience (Rosen, 2002). Paracervical blocks are associated with fetal bradycardia and are seldom used since the introduction of epidural analgesia (Leeman, Fontaine & King, et al, 2003a; Rosen, 2002).

Non-Pharmacological Pain Management Strategies

Expert labor nurses develop a repertoire of skills to assist women with management of labor pain. Comfort measures include ambulation, hydrotherapy, deep breathing, pelvic rocking, rocking on a birthing ball, massage, hynobirthing, intradermal water blocks, and acupressure/acupuncture (Hardin & Buckner, 2004; Harris, 1999; Leeman, Fontaine, King, et al, 2003b). Such strategies provide effective alternatives to pharmacological methods and are discussed in systematic reviews (Simkin & O'Hara, 2002; Smith, Collins & Crowther, 2003; Simkin & O'Hara, 2002). For example, in a Cochrane review, "[the woman's] ability to move freely and assume a variety of positions while pushing work in concert with [natural endorphins]" (Torvaldsen, Roberts, Bell, et al, 2004). One nurse reported,

> My bag of tricks is based on twenty years experience...getting patients out of bed, foot and back massages, the birthing ball, and the shower or tub. Of course you need to give positive feedback too, so they will know you think they are doing well (James, Simpson & Knox, 2003, p. 818).

Implications for Clinical Practice

According to Tumblin and Simkin (2001), a systematic review of pain and women's satisfaction with childbirth (Hodnett, 2002), and a Cochrane review which evaluated 15 studies, (Hodnett, Gates, Hofmeyr, et al, 2004), as care providers and birthing centers seek to fulfill women's expectations of birth, women report positive childbirth experiences, satisfaction with pain management, and satisfaction with their birth. The influence of pain,

pain relief, and medical interventions is not as powerful as the attitudes, skills, and behaviors of caregivers (Hodnett, 2002). Lothian (1993) noted that women who experience a supportive birthing environment were more likely to chose to give birth without medication. Childbirth has become medicalized (Riessman, 1983) over time with the application of technology such as continuous fetal monitoring, epidural anesthesia, administration of intravenous fluids, oxytocin induction and augmentation, routine episiotomy, and instrumentally assisted vaginal births (Miesnik & Stringer, 2002)

The use of technology should be balanced with the provision of physical, emotional, and spiritual support (Miesnik & Stringer, 2002). In addition to professional support, there is a growing movement to have support from doulas (Bianchi & Adams, 2004; Meyer, Arnold & Pascali-Bonaro, 2001) as well as fathers and extended female members (Pascali-Bonaro & Kroeger, 2004; Pascoe, 1993).

In a study of Chinese women, women whose husbands were present in the birthing room used significantly higher levels of analgesia than those whose husbands were not present (Ip, 2000). This appears to give evidence that husbands also need professional help and role modeling in order to provide support for the laboring woman (Thomassen, Lundwall, Wiger, et al, 2003).

Encouragement, demonstration of respect, and conveying a sense of shared power is so important (Hogberg, 1994; Matthews & Callister, 2004). Women should be empowered to give birth (Hogberg, 1994). One nurse said, *"I always tell my patients, 'you can do this. We can do this together"* (James, Simpson & Knox, 2003, p. 819). Kennedy and Shannon (2004) also suggest the importance of belief and trust in a woman's strength. A nurse midwife participating in their study said,

> Listening and being able to help a woman find her strength and use her strength [is so important]. I think giving birth can lend a lot of strength to women that have not done anything successful in their life, or maybe don't feel like they have (p. 558).

Supportive care articulated by professional organizations includes the dimensions of physical care, emotional care, the provision of education, and advocacy (AWHONN, 2001, 2002). World Health Organization principles of promoting normal birth include providing continuous emotional and physical support during labor (Lothian, 2002). While the effectiveness of nurses as providers of support during labor and birth has not been demonstrated to be superior to continuous support by others (Hodnett, Lowe, Hannah, et al, 2002), there is evidence of positive psychosocial and physiological outcomes.

Over two decades of research have documented positive outcomes from support such as shorter labors, less use of analgesia/anesthesia, fewer instrumental vaginal births or cesarean births, decreased oxytocin, and increased satisfaction have been demonstrated (Sauls, 2002; Scott, Klaus & Klaus, 1999).

Gagnon and Waghorn evaluated one to one labor support of first time mothers receiving oxytocin (1999). In a study using the Bryanton Adaptation of the Nursing Support in Labor Questionnaire (BANSILQ) (Bryanton, Fraser-Davey & Sullivan, 1994). Items scored highest by childbearing women were "makes me feel cared about as an individual" and "treated me with respect." The item, "gave me pain medication" was only ranked 17th out of 25th (Corbett & Callister, 2000) which provides evidence that analgesia was not the major consideration for these women but rather was superseded by a supportive relationship.

Even the smallest demonstrations of support and caring can make a tremendous difference: a kind word, touch, eye contact, and actively listening (Hunter, 2002). Simkin (2000) has identified a toolkit of supportive strategies that can be easily implemented by busy clinicians. This can be done as care interventions are integrated with supportive care (AWHONN, 2002; Miltner, 2002). In a study of the effects of epidural analgesia/anesthesia, researchers concluded that,

> It is quite alarming to see how nurses and physicians rely on epidural analgesia in labor. Many nurses who practice in institutions where it is the preferred analgesia have lost their clinical ability to coach and assist through labor without an epidural. Sometimes when a woman demands an epidural [what] she may really...need is encouragement, position changes, touching, and a caring attitude from her caregiver (Thorpe, McNitt & Leppert, 1990, p. 158).

Simkin's Pain Medications Preference Scale (2000) can be utilized to link assessment of preferences about pharmacologic pain relief to support by caregivers. Manogin and associates (2000) developed a Caring Behavior Assessment to define the most helpful behaviors from the perspectives of childbearing women. Miltner (2002) developed a Supportive Surveillance Model of Care (2002) which includes not only ensuring the physical well being of the mother and the fetus/newborn but also maximizing the psychosocial well being of not only mother and child but the family as well. It has been recommended that labor support certification be required for labor nurses just as certification in fetal monitoring is often required (Sauls, 2002). A number of factors influence the ability of the labor nurse to provide continuous support, including the nursing shortage, other limited health care resources, staffing ratios, organization mission and values, management support, unit protocols, unit culture, and staff attitudes (AWHONN, 2000; Davies & Hodnett, 2001; Marmor & Krol, 2002).

There are often differences identified in perceptions of labor pain between women and professionals attending their birth, with caregivers underestimating pain intensity at levels that women described as severe (Baker, Ferguson, Roach, et al, 2001). In addition, opinions of caregivers range from "those who feel that pain is a natural part of childbirth and it's experience provides powerful lessons, to those who believe that childbirth pain is not different from pain from all illness or injury and that it is inhumane to let laboring women suffer" (Grainger & McCool, 1998, p. 250). Some caregivers conclude that women whose stated preference is to be unmedicated are "either martyrs or misinformed" (Hodnett, 2002, p. S170). This is affirmed by Lowe, "the clinician, in the interest of helping, cannot understanding why some women choose to persevere and labor without analgesia in the face of pain" (Lowe, 2002, p. S22).

One childbearing woman described what advocacy meant, *"The nurses are supportive of what you want, who you are, and how you want to do things"* (Mackey & Stepans, 1994, p. 416). Laboring women are vulnerable and less able to advocate for themselves, and particularly susceptible to the exercise of verbal and non-verbal power from their caregivers which may be either positive or negative (Sinivaara, Suominen, Routasalo, et al, 2004). This vulnerability was expressed by one woman who had recently given birth,

> Because of the position a laboring woman is in, you're at everybody's [mercy]. It's such tiny little things that can affect you in such large ways. They can affect your labor. I mean, one

> positive word or touch can make, for me, a grand difference in how what's gonna happen in the next minutes or hours is going to turn out (VandeVusse, 1999, p. 182).

Sinivaara and associates (2004) also concluded that only 29% of childbearing women in their study felt that the decision regarding pain relief was made solely by her. One woman expressed willingness to relinquish control to her caregivers,

> If they say to me, you know, "Would you like an epidural?" If I feel that I don't need one, I'm going to say, "No." But if then they say, "We think it might be a good idea if you had one," I'd probably say, "Oh, go on then," you know? Because in the long run they're the experts, you know" (Weaver, 1998, p.85).

The process of labor and birth is dynamic, as are the woman's sense of and need for control which may vary significantly. According to Weaver (1998, p. 93), "A woman's perception of control and thus her willingness to make decisions will ebb and flow throughout her labor." Because of this, a birth plan is helpful so the woman can concentrate on the labor process rather than continually making decisions (Bowers, 2002).

Antepartum education of women is essential. Hospital based prenatal offerings are largely an orientation to institutional policies and procedures with an emphasis on compliance with hospital regimes rather than focusing on the needs of the women (Armstrong, 2000). Education of women about pain management options and their risks and benefits are essential for informed consent (Lowe, 2004). The Journal of Midwifery and Women's Health (2004) has developed patient education material to share with women on pain during childbirth. Websites for women provide consumer friendly information about pain management during childbirth which is updated regularly based on the latest credible evidence.

The provision of culturally competent care for childbearing women has becoming increasingly emphasized in the delivery of health care (Callister, 2001, 2005), since it is projected by 2050 that diverse cultural groups will constitute 48% of the population (http://www.quickfacts.census.gov). Pain management strategies for culturally diverse women should include awareness and knowledge, skills, and sensitivity. Health care providers should seek to develop a common vocabulary for exploring the pain of childbirth and the provision of comfort (Jimenez, 1996, 1998).

Table 2. Childbirth Pain and Pain Relief Websites

Childbirth.org: Pain and pain relief methods
http://www.childbirth.org/articles/labor/painrelief.html
Maternity Center Association
http://www.maternitywise.org/mw/topics/laborsupport/
http://www.maternitywise.org/mw/topics/pain/tips.html.
Doulas of North America
http://www.dona.org

"Finding a fit" with the caregiver is also essential, contributing to better pain management and satisfaction with the birth experience (Callister, 1994). Health beliefs and perceptions of women with either obstetrician or certified nurse midwife (CNM) caregivers differed, and women with obstetricians had significantly higher rates of epidural anesthesia. Women with CNM caregivers wanted to feel a sense of control and the ability to influence care decisions (Callister, 1995).

Since the 1930's, there has been an increasing stream of women's accounts of childbirth being published (Cosslet, 1994). Women are accessing birth stories on a number of websites, and such electronic connectedness fosters integration of the birth experience into women's lives (Farley & Widmann, 2001). Listening to the voices of women through accessing birth stories is an important clinical intervention (Callister, 2004; Gamble & Creedy, 2004; Inglis, 2002; Kalmen & Ancheta, 1997; Lothian, 2003; McKenzie-McHarg, 2004; Steele & Beadle, 2003; Wessely, Rose & Bisson, 2000).

Implications for Research

Since research is so limited on the pain experience of culturally diverse women, further inquiry is indicated in order to foster culturally competent health care (Callister, 2005). More studies are needed of women regarding preferences for an unmedicated birth who subsequently had medicated births building on the work of Goldberg, Cohen and Lieberman (1999) as well as Carlton, Callister and Stoneman (2005) and the influence of caregivers on those practices (Grannger & McCool (1998). A tool has been developed to elicit beliefs about pain (Lasch, 2000) which may be tested in women giving birth. Because of the documented relationship between feelings of control and childbirth pain, a tool has been developed with dimensions include informational control, a sense of control in decision making, and personal control of emotions and behaviors which needs further testing (McCrea, Wright & Stringer, 2000) so that measurement of nursing support can be refined (Gale, Fothergill-Bourbonnais & Chamberlain, 2001)

Replication of the work of Ferber and associates (2005) using the 13 item Pain Catastrophizing Scale (PCS) developed by Sullivan, Bishop and Pivic (1995) as an assessment tool for laboring woman in conjunction with the Visual Analog Scale (VAS) would be of value.

Childbirth accounts for 12% of hospital admissions, and is the most common cause of such admissions (Centers for Disease Control, 2000). Facilitating appropriate pain management with consideration of multiple complex variables including continuous support is essential to ensure positive outcomes from giving birth.

Acknowledgements

Appreciation is expressed for funding from the Brigham Young University College of Nursing, and Office for Research and Creative Activity; Council for International Exchange of Scholars (Fulbright Scholarship); Kennedy Center for International Studies; Sigma Theta Tau International Iota Iota Chapter; and the Women's Research Institute; and to the childbearing women who shared their voices.

REFERENCES

Aldrich, S. & Eccleston, C. (2000). Making sense of everyday pain. *Social Science and Medicine, 50,* 1631-1641.

Armstrong, E.M. (2000). Lessons in control: Prenatal education in the hospital. *Social Problems, 47*(4), 583-605.

Association of Womens Health, Obstetric, and Neonatal Nurses (AWHONN). (2000). *Professional Nursing Support of Laboring Women. Clinical Position Statement.* Washington, D.C.: AWHONN. http://www.awhonn.org Retrieved February 11, 2004.

Association of Womens Health, Obstetric, and Neonatal Nurses (AWHONN). (2001). *Nursing Care of the Woman Receiving Regional Analgesia/Anesthesia in Labor. Evidence Based Clinical Practice Guideline.* Washington, D.C.: AWHONN.

Association of Womens Health, Obstetric, and Neonatal Nurses (AWHONN). (2002). *Nursing Management of Second Stage Labor.* Washington, D.C.: AWHONN.

Baker, A., Ferguson, S.A., Roach, G.D. & Dawson, D. (2001). Perceptions of labour pain by mothers and their attending midwives. *Journal of Advanced Nursing, 35* (2), 171-179.

Beck, C.T. (2004a). Birth trauma: In the eye of the beholder. *Nursing Research, 53*(1), 28-35.

Beck, C.T. (2004b). Post-traumatic stress disorder due to childbirth. *Nursing Research, 53*(4), 216-224.

Bergum, V. (1989). *Woman to Mother: A Transformation.* Granby, Maryland: Bergin & Garvey.

Bianchi, A.L. & Adams, E.D. (2004). Doulas, labor support, and nurses. *International Journal of Childbirth Education, 19*(4), 24-30.

Bowers, B.B. (2002). Mothers' experiences of labor support: Exploration of qualitative research. *Journal of Obstetric, Gynecologic, and Neonatal Nursing, 31*(6), 511-521.

Bricker, L. & Lavender T. (2002). Parenteral opioids for labor pain relief: A systematic review. *American Journal of Obstetrics and Gynecology, 186*(Suppl 5), 94-109. http://www.maternitywise.org/prof/pain

Bryanton, J., Fraser-Davey, H. & Sullivan, P. (1994). Women's perceptions of nursing support during labor. *Journal of Obstetric, Gynecologic, and Neonatal Nursing, 23* (8), 638-644.

Callister, L.C., Lauri, S. & Vehvilainen-Julkunen, K. (2000). A description of birth in Finland. *MCN: The American Journal of Maternal Child Nursing, 25*(3), 146-150.

Callister, L.C. (1995). Beliefs and perceptions of childbearing women choosing different primary health care providers. *Clinical Nursing Research, 4,* 168-180.

Callister, L.C., Semenic, S. & Foster, J.C. (1999). Cultural and spiritual meanings of Childbirth: Orthodox Jewish and Mormon women. *Journal of Holistic Nursing, 17*(3), 280-295.

Callister, L.C. (2003). Cultural influences on pain perception and behaviors. *Home Health Care Management and Practice, 15*(3), 207-211.

Callister, L.C. (1995). Cultural meanings of childbirth. *Journal of Obstetric, Gynecologic, and Neonatal Nursing, 24,* 327-351.

Callister, L.C., Vehvailinen-Julkunen, K. & Lauri, S. (1996). Cultural perceptions of childbirth: A cross-cultural comparison of childbearing women. *Journal of Holistic Nursing, 14*(1), 66-78.

Callister, L.C. (2001). Culturally competent care of women and newborns: Attitudes, knowledge, and skills. *Journal of Obstetric, Gynecologic, and Neonatal Nursing,30 (2),* 209-215.

Callister, L.C. (1994). Finding a fit: Choice of a health care provider by childbearing women. *Clinical Consultations in Obstetrics and Gynecology, 6*(4), 252-257.

Callister, L.C. & Vega, R. (1998). Giving birth: Guatemalan women's voices. *Journal of Obstetric, Gynecologic, and Neonatal Nursing, 27*(3), 289-295.

Callister, L.C., Vehvailinen-Julkunen, K. &Lauri, S. (2001). Giving birth: Perceptions of Finnish childbearing women. *MCN: The American Journal of Maternal Child Nursing, 26*(1), 28-32.

Callister, L.C., Getmanenko, N., Garvrish, N., Eugenevna, M.O., Vladiminov, A., Turkina, N., & Lassetter, N., (2006). Giving birth: The voices of Russian women. *MCN: The American Journal of Maternal Child Nursing*, in review.

Callister, L.C. (2006). Integrating cultural beliefs and practice into the care of childbearing women. In K.R.Simpson & P.A. Creehan (Eds). *Perinatal Nursing* (3rd edition), Philadelphia: Lippincott, in press.

Callister, L.C. (2004). Making meaning: Women's birth narratives. *Journal of Obstetric, Gynecologic, and Neonatal Nursing, 33*(4), 508-518.

Callister, L.C. (1992). The meaning of the childbirth experience to the Mormon woman. *Journal of Perinatal Education, 1*(1), 50-57.

Callister, L.C., Khalaf, I., Semenic, S., Kartchner, & Vehvilainen-Julkunen, K. (2003). The pain of childbirth: Perceptions of culturally diverse women. *Pain Management Nursing, 4*(4), 145-154.

Callister, L.C. (1993). The role of the nurse in childbirth: Perceptions of the childbearing woman. *Clinical Nurse Specialist, 7*(6), 288-293.

Callister, L.C. (2005). What do we know from the literature about cultural competence in the care of women and children? *MCN: The American Journal of Maternal Child Nursing, 30*(6), 4-12.

Capik, L.K. (1998). Health beliefs of childbearing women: The choice of epidurals for pain management. *The Journal of Perinatal Education, 7*(3), 7-17.

Carlton, T., Callister, L.C. & Stoneman, E. (2005). Decision making in laboring Women: Ethical issues for perinatal nurses. *Journal of Perinatal and Neonatal Nursing, 19*(2), 145-154.

Caton, D., Frolich, M.A. & Euliano, T.Y. (2002). Anesthesia for childbirth: Controversy and change. *American Journal of Obstetrics and Gynecology, 186*(5 Suppl), S-25-30. http://www.marternitywise.org/prof/pain

Caton, D., Corry, M.P., Frigoletto, F.D., Hopkins, D.P., Lieberman, E., Mayberry, L., Rooks, J.P., Rosenfield, A., Sakala, C., Simkin, P. & Young, D. (2002). The nature and management of labor pain. *American Journal of Obstetrics and Gynecology, 186*(5 Suppl), S1-15. http://www.maternitywise.org/prof/pain

Centers for Disease Control. (2002). *National Center for Health Statistics/Births/Natalities.* http://www.cdc.gov/nchs/fastats/births/htm

Corbett, C.A. & Callister, L.C. (2000). Nursing support during labor. *Clinical Nursing Research, 9*(1), 70-83.

Cosslet, T. (1994). *Women Writing Childbirth.* Manchester, NY: Manchester University Press.

Creedy, D.K., Shochet, I.M. & Horsfall, J. (2000). Childbirth and the development of acute trauma symptoms: Incidence and contributing factors. *Birth, 27*(2), 104-111.

Czarnocka, J. & Slade, P. (2000). Prevalence and predictors of post-traumatic stress symptoms following childbirth. *British Journal of Clinical Psychology, 39,* 35-51.

Davies, B.L. & Hodnett, E. (2002). Labor support: Nurses' self-efficacy and views about factors influencing implementation. *Journal of Obstetric, Gynecologic, and Neonatal Nursing, 31*(1), 48-56.

Davis-Floyd, R. (1986). Afterword. In R.B Star. *The Healing Power of Birth.* Austin, Texas: Star Publishing.

Enkin, M., Keierse, M.J.N.C., Neilson, J., Crowther, C., Duley, L., Hodnett, E. & Hofmeyr, J. (2000). *A guide to effective care in pregnancy and childbirth.* New York: Oxford University Press.

Farley, C. & Widmann, S. (2001). The value of birth stories. *International Journal of Childbirth Education, 16*(3), 22-25.

Ferber, S.G., Granot, M. & Zimmer, E.Z. (2005). Catastrophizing labor pain compromises later maternity adjustments. *American Journal of Obstetrics and Gynecology, 192,* 826-831.

Fowles, E.R. (1998). Labor concerns of women two months after delivery. *Birth, 25*(4), 235-240.

Gagnon, A.J. & Waghorn, K. (1999). One to one labor support of nulliparous women stimulated with oxytocin. *Journal of Obstetric, Gynecologic, and Neonatal Nursing, 28*(4), 371-376.

Gale, J., Fothergill-Bourbonnais, F. & Chamberlain, M. (2001). Measuring nursing support during childbirth. *MCN: The American Journal of Maternal Child Nursing, 26*(5), 264-271.

Gamble, J. & Creedy, D. (2004). Content and processes of postpartum counseling after a distressing birth experience. *Birth, 31*(3), 213-218.

Goldberg, A.B., Cohen, A. & Lieberman, E. (1999). Nulliparas' preferences for epidural analgesia: Their effects on actual use in labor. *Birth, 26*(3), 139-143.

Goodman, P. Mackey, M.M. & Tavakoli, A.S. (2004). Factors related to childbirth satisfaction. *Journal of Advanced Nursing, 46*(2), 212-219.

Graninger, E.M. & McCool, W.P. (1998). Nurse-midwives use of and attitudes toward epidural analgesia. *Journal of Nurse Midwifery, 43*(4), 250-260..

Green, J.M. & Baston, H.A. (2003). Feeling in control during labor: Concepts, correlates, and consequences. *Birth, 30*(4), 235-247.

Green, J.M., Coupland, V.A. & Kitzinger, J.V. (1998). *Great Expectations: A Prospective Study of Women's Expectations and Experiences of Childbirth.* Cheshire, England: Books for Midwives Press.

Hardin, A.M. & Buckner, E.B. (2004). Characteristics of a positive experience for women who have unmedicated childbirth. *The Journal of Perinatal Education, 13*(4), 10-16.

Harris, K.T. (1999). Hydrotherapy: An alternative method for relieving labor pain. *Mother Baby Journal, 4*(5), 15-22.

Hodnett, E.D., Gates, S., Hofmeyr, G.J. Sakala, C. (2004). Continuous support for women during childbirth (Cochrane Review). In the *Cochrane Library* (2). Chichester, UK: John Wiley & Sons.

Hodnett, E., Lowe, N., Hannah, A., Willian, B., Steens, J., Weston, A., Ohlsson, A., Gafni, H., Muir, T, Myhr, T. & Stremler, R. (2002). Effectiveness of nurses as providers of birth labor support. *The Journal of the American Medical Association, 288*(1), 1373-1381.

Hodnett, E.D. (2002). Pain and women's satisfaction with the experience of childbirth: A systematic review. *American Journal of Obstetrics and Gynecology, 186*(5 Suppl), S160-172. Available at http://www.maternitywise.org/prof/pain

Hogberg, L. (1994). Empowering women to give birth. *Journal of Perinatal Education, 3* (3), 43-45.

Howell, C.J. (2004). Epidural versus non-epidural analgesia for pain relief in labor (Cochrane Review). In the *Cochrane Library* (2). Chichester, UK: John Wiley & Sons.

Hunter, J.P. (2002). Being with woman: A guiding concept for the care of laboring women. *Journal of Obstetric, Gynecologic, and Neonatal Nursing, 31*(6), 650-657.

Inglis, S. (2002). Accessing a debriefing service following birth. *Journal of Midwifery, 10*(6), 368-371.

Ip, W.Y. (2000). Chinese husbands' presence during labour. *International Journal of Nursing Practice, 6,* 89-96.

James, D.C., Simpson, K.R. & Knox, G.E. (2003). How do expert labor nurses view their role? *Journal of Obstetric, Gynecologic, and Neonatal Nursing, 32*(6), 814-823.

Jimenez, S.L.M. (1996). Establishing a common vocabulary for exploring issues of pain and comfort. *The Journal of Perinatal Education, 5,* 54-57.

Jimenez, S.L.M. (1998). Pain and comfort assessment: The key to effective pain management. *The Journal of Perinatal Education, 7*(1), 35-38.

Jimenez, S.L.M. (2000). Supportive strategies for childbirth. In F.H. Nichols & S.S. Humenick (Eds). *Childbirth Education: Practice, Research, and Theory* (2nd edition), pp. 155-177. Philadelphia: W.B. Saunders.

Joint Commission for the Accreditation of Health Care Organizations.(2003). *Joint Commission Resources: 2004 Comprehensive Accreditation Manual for Hospitals.* Oakbrook Terrace, IL: JCAHO.

Johnson T. & Callister, L.C. (in review), Giving birth at home in The Netherlands.

Journal of Midwifery and Women's Health. (2004). Pain during childbirth. *Journal of Midwifery and Women's Health, 49*(6), 553-554. Pain education handout.

Kalmen, B. & Ancheta, R. (1997). Back talk: Debriefing new mothers. *Childbirth Instructor, 1997 1st Quarter,* 40.

Kanna, S., Jamison, R.N. & Datta, S. (2001). Maternal satisfaction and pain control in women electing natural childbirth. *Regional Anesthesia and Pain Medicine, 26*(5), 468-472.

Kardong-Edgren, S. (1999). Is it time to change the paradigm? *Journal of Obstetric, Gynecologic, and Neonatal Nursing, 28*(5), 477-479.

Kartchner, R. & Callister, L.C. (1997). Cultural meanings of childbirth: The voices of childbearing women. *Journal of Holistic Nursing, 21*(2), 100-116.

Kennedy, H.P. & Shannon, M.T. (2004). Keeping birth normal: Research findings on midwifery care during childbirth. *Journal of Obstetric, Gynecologic, and Neonatal Nursing, 33*(5), 554-560.

Khalaf, I. & Callister, L.C. (1997). Cultural meanings of childbirth: Muslim women living in Jordan. *Journal of Holistic Nursing, 15*(4), 373-387.

Lasch, K.E. (2000). Culture, pain, and culturally sensitive pain care. *Pain Management Nursing, 1*(3), Suppl 1, 16-22.

Lavender, T., Walkinshaw, S.A. & Walton, I. (1999). A prospective study of women's views of factors contributing to a positive birth experience. *Midwifery, 15,* 40-46.

Leeman, L., Fontaine, P., King, V., Klein, M.C. & Ratcliffe, S. (2003). Management of labor pain: Promoting patient choice. *American Family Physician, 68*(6), 1023-1024, 1033-1034.

Leeman, L.., Fontaine, P., King, V., Klein, M.C. & Ratcliffe, S. (2003b). The nature and management of labor pain. Part I: Nonpharmacologic pain relief. *American Family Physician, 68*(6), 1109-1112.

Leeman, L., Fontaine, P., King, V., Klein, M.C. & Ratcliffe, S. (2003a). The nature and management of labor pain: Part II. Pharmacologic pain relief. *American Family Physician, 68*(6), 1115-1120.

Leighton, B.L. & Halpern, S.H. (2002). The effects of epidural analgesia on labor, maternal, and neonatal outcomes: A systematic review. *American Journal of Obstetrics and Gynecology, 186*(Suppl 5), 69-77.

Lieberman, E. & O'Donoghue, C. (2002). Unintended effects of epidural analgesia during labor: A systematic review. *American Journal of Obstetrics and Gynecology, 186* (5 Suppl), S31-68. http://www.maternitywise.org/prof/pain

Lothian, J.A. (2002). Listening to mothers: The first national United States survey of women's childbearing experiences. *The Journal of Perinatal Education, 12*(1), vi-vii.

Lothian, J.A. (2002). Promoting, protecting, and supporting normal birth. *The Journal of Perinatal Education, 11*(3), vii-x.

Lothian, J.A. (1993). Why do women chose epidurals? *Journal of Perinatal Education, 2*(2), 9-10.

Lowe, N. (2004). Context and process of informed consent for pharmacologic strategies in labor pain care. *Journal of Midwifery and Womens Health, 49*(3), 250-259.

Lowe, N. (2000).Self-efficacy and childbirth fears in nulliparous pregnant women. *Journal of Psychosomatic Obstetrics and Gynecology, 21,* 219-224.

Lowe, N.K. (2002). The nature of labor pain. *American Journal of Obstetrics and Gynecology, 186*(5 Suppl), S16-24. http://www.maternitywise.org/prof/pain

Luckmann, J. (1999). *Transcultural Communication in Nursing.* Albany NY: Delmar.

Lundgren, I., Berg, M. & Lindmark, G. (2003). Is the childbirth experience improved by a birth plan? *Journal of Midwifery and Womens Health, 48,* 322-328.

Lundgren, I. & Dahlber, C.K. (1998). Women's experience of pain during childbirth. *Midwifery, 14*(2), 105-110.

Maclean, L.I., McDermott, M.R. & May, C.P. (2000). Method of delivery and subjective distress: Women's emotional responses to childbirth practices. *Journal of Reproductice and Infant Psychology, 18*(2), 153-162.

McCrea, H. & Wright, M.E. (1999). Satisfaction in childbirth and perceptions of personal control in pain relief during labour. *Journal of Advanced Nursing, 29*(4), 877-884.

McCrea, H., Wright, M. & Stringer, M. (2000). The development of a scale to assess control in pain management during labor. *Journal of Reproductive and Infant Psychology, 18*(2), 105-115.

McCrea, B.H. & Wright, M.E. (1999). Satisfaction in childbirth and perceptions of personal control in pain relief during labor. *Journal of Advanced Nursing, 29*(4), 877-884.

McKenzie-McHarg, K. (2004). Traumatic birth: Understanding predictors, triggers, and counseling process is essential to treatment. *Birth, 31*((3), 219-221.

Mander, R. (1998). *Pain in Childbearing and It's Control.* Oxford, ENG: Blackwell.

Mander, R. (2000). The meanings of labor pain or the layers of an onion? A woman oriented view. *Journal of Reproductive and Infant Psychology, 18*(2), 133-141.

Manogin, T.W., Bechtel, G.A. & Rami, J.S. (2000). Caring behaviors by nurses: Women's perceptions during childbirth. *Journal of Obstetric, Gynecologic, and Neonatal Nursing, 29*(2), 153-157.

Marmor, T.R. & Krol, D.M. (2002). Labor pain management in the United States: understanding patterns and the issue of choice. *American Journal of Obstetrics and Gynecology, 186*(Suppl 5), 173-180.

Maternity Center Association. (2002). *Labor Pain Initiative.* http://www.maternitywise.org/ *prof/pain/values*

Matthews, R. & Callister, L.C. (2004). Childbearing women's perceptions of nursing care that promotes dignity. *Journal of Obstetric, Gynecologic, and Neonatal Nursing, 33*(4), 498-507.

Mayberry, L.J., Clemmens, D. & De, A. (2002). Epidural analgesia side effects: Co-interventions, and care of women during childbirth: A systematic review. *American Journal of Obstetrics and Gynecology, 186*(Suppl 5), 81-93. http://www. maternitywise.org/prof/pain

Melender, H.L. & Lauri, S. (2001). Security associated with pregnancy and childbirth—Experiences of pregnant women. *Journal of Psychosomatic Obstetrics and Gynecology, 22,* 229-239.

Meyer, B., Arnold, J., Pascali-Bonaro, D. (2001). Social support by doulas during labor and the early postpartum period. *Hospital Physician, September,* 57-65.

Mesnik, S.R. & Stringer, M. (2002). Technology in the birthing room. *Nursing Clinics of North America, 37*(4), 781-793.

Miltner, R.S. (2002). More than support: Nursing interventions provided to women in labor. *Journal of Obstetric, Gynecologic, and Neonatal Nursing, 31*(6), 753-761.

Nayak, S., Shiflett, S.C., Eshun, S. & Levine, F.M. (2000). Culture and gender effects on pain beliefs and the prediction of pain tolerance. *Cross Cultural Research, 34,* 135-141.

Niven, C.A. & Gijsbers, K. (1996). Perinatal pain. In C.A. Niven & A. Walker (Eds). *The psychology of reproduction, 2,* 131-147. Oxford: Butterworth Heinemann.

Niven, C.A. & Murphy-Black, T. (2000). Memory for labor pain: A review of the literature. *Birth, 27*(4), 244-255.

Nystedt, A., Hogberg, U. & Lundman, B. (2005). The negative birth experience of prolonged labour: A case-referent study. *Journal of Clinical Nursing, 14*(5), 579-587.

Pascali-Bonaro, D. & Kroeger, M. (2004). Continuous female companionship during childbirth: A critical resource in times of stress or calm. *Journal of Midwifery and Women's Health, 49*(4), 19-27.

Pascoe, J. (1993). Social support during labor and duration of labor: A community based study. *Public health Nursing, 10*(2), 97-99.

Petree, B. & Walsch, L.V. (2001). Maintenance of comfort and management of pain. In L.V. Walsch. *Midwifery: Community Based Care During the Chidlbearing Year,* pp. 245-262.

Poore, M. & Foster, J.C. (1985). Epidural and no epidural anesthesia: Differences between mothers and their experiences of birth. *Birth, 12*(4), 205-212.

Riessman, C.K. (1983). Women and medicalization: A new perspective. *Social Policy, Summer,* 3-18.

Rosen, M.A. (2002). Nitrous oxide for relief of labor pain: A systematic review. *American Journal of Obstetrics and Gynecology, 186*(Suppl5), 110-126. http://www.maternitywise.org/prof/pain

Rosen, M.A. (2002). Paracervical block for labor analgesia: A brief historic review. *American Journal of Obstetrics and Gynecology, 186*(Suppl 5), 127-130. http://www.maternitywise.org/prof/pain

Salmon, R., Miller, R. & Drew, N.C. (1990). Women's anticipation and experience of childbirth: The interdependence of fulfillment, unpleasantness, and pain. *British Journal of Medical Psychology, 63*(Part 3), 255-259.

Sauls, D.J. (2002). Effects of labor support on mothers, babies, and birth outcomes. *Journal of Obstetric, Gynecologic, and Neonatal Nursing, 31*(6), 733-741.

Schrim, H., Tobi, L.T.W., Vandenberg, L. (2002). Low use of medication in home deliveries in the Netherlands. *International Journal of Obstetrics and Gynecology, 79,* 5-9.

Scott, K.D., Klaus, P.H. & Klaus, M.H. (1999). The obstetrical and postpartum benefits of continuous support during childbirth. *Journal of Women's Health and Gender Based Medicine, 8*(10), 1257-1264.

Semenic, S.E., Callister, L.C., & Feldman, P. (2004). Giving birth: The voices of Orthodox Jewish women living in Canada. *Journal of Obstetrics, Gynecologic, and Neonatal Nursing, 33*(1), 80-87.

Simkin, P. (1991). Just another day in a woman's life? Women's long-term perceptions of their first birth experience. Part I. *Birth, 18,* 203-210.

Simkin, P. & O'Hara, M.A. (2002). Nonpharmacologic relief of pain during labor: Systematic review of five methods. *American Journal of Obstetrics and Gynecology, 186*(Suppl 5), 131-159.

Simkin, P. (2002). Supportive care during labor: A guide for busy nurses. *Journal of Obstetric, Gynecologic, and Neonatal Nurses, 31*(6), 721-732.

Simkin, P. (2000). *The Birth Partner.* Boston: Harvard Common Press.

Sinivaara, M., Suominen, T., Routasalo, P. & Hupli, M. (2004). How delivery ward staff exercise power over women in commmunciation. *Journal of Advanced Nursing, 46*(1), 33-41.

Smith, C.A., Collins, C.T., Cya, A.M. & Crowther, C.A. (2003). Complementary and alternative therapies for pain management in labour. (Cochrane Review). In the *Cochrane Library*(3). Chichester, UK: John Wiley & Sons.

Soet, J.E., Breck, G.A. & Dilorio, C. (2003). Prevalence and predictors of women's experience of psychological trauma during childbirth. *Birth, 30*(1), 36-46.

Steele, A.M. & Beadle, M. (2003). A survey of postnatal debriefing. *Journal of Advanced Nursing, 43*(2), 130-136.

Sullivan, M.J.L., Bishop, S. & Pivic, J. (1995). The pain catastrophizing scale: Development and validation. *Psychological Assessment, 7*, 524-732.

Thacker, S.B. & Stroup, D.F. (2002). Methods and interpretation in systematic reviews: Commentary on two parallel reviews of epidural analgesia during labor. *American Journal of Obstetrics and Gynecology, 186*(Suppl 5), 78-80.

Thomassen, P., Lundwall, M., Wiger, E., Wollin, L., Uvnas-Moberg, K. (2003). Doula: A new concept in obstetrics. *Larkartidningen, 100,* 4268-4271.

Thorpe, J.A., McNitt, J.D. & Leppert, P.C. (1990). The effects of epidural anesthesia. *Birth, 17*(3), 157-162.

Torvaldsen, S., Roberts, C.L., Bell, J.C. & Rayne-Greenow, C.H. (2004). Discontinuation of epidural analgesia late in labour for reducing the adverse delivery outcomes associated with epidural analgesia (Cochrane Review). *The Cochrane Library (4).*

Tumblin, A. & Simkin, P. (2001). Pregnant women's perceptions of their nurse's role during labor and delivery. *Birth, 28,* 52-56.

Van der Hulst, L.A.M., van Teijlingen, E.R., Bonsel, G.J., Eskes, M. & Bleker, O.P. (2004). Does a pregnant woman's intended place of birth influence her attitudes toward and occurrence of obstetric interventions? *Birth, 31*(1), 28-33.

VandeVusse, L. (1999). The essential forces of labor revisited: 13 P's reported in women's stories. *MCN: The American Journal of Maternal Child Nursing, 24*(4), 176-184.

Waldenstrom, U., Hildingsson, I., Rubertsson, C. & Radestad, I. (2004). A negative birth experience: Prevalence and risk factors in a national sample. *Birth, 31*(1), 17-27.

Waldenstrom, U. (1999). Experience of labor and birth in 1111 women. *Journal of Psychosomatic Research, 5,* 471-482.

Waldenstrom, U., Berg, I.M., Olsson, B., Skold, M. & Wall, S. (1996). The childbirth experience: A study of 295 new mothers. *Birth, 25*(3), 144-153.

Waldenstrom, U. (2004). Why do some women change their opinion about childbirth over time? *Birth, 31*(2), 102-107.

Weaver, J. (1998). Choice, control, and decision-making in labour. In S. Clement (Ed). *Psychological Perspectives on Pregnancy and Childbirth,* pp. 81-99. Edinburgh: Churchill Livingstone.

Weber, S.F. (1996). Cultural aspects of pain in childbearing women. *Journal of Obstetric, Gynecologic, and Neonatal Nursing, 25*(1), 67-72.

Wessely, S., Rose, S. & Bisson, J.A. (2000). A systematic review of brief psychological interventions ("debriefing") for the treatment of immediate trauma related symptoms and the prevention of post traumatic stress disorder. In the *Cochrane Library, Volume 4.* Oxford: Update Software.

Wright, M.E., McCrea, H., Stringer, M. & Murphy-Black, T. (2000). Personal control in pain relief during labour. *Journal of Advanced Nursing, 32*(5), 1168-1177.

INDEX

A

B

C

D

E

F

G

H

I

J

K

L

M

N

O

P

T